LIVING IN REVERSE

How reversing diabetes and obesity
can help you create sustainable lives
and sustainable communities

TED SCHIERER PH.D.

Published by JETT Publishing

8350 EP True Parkway Unit 1201
West Des Moines, Iowa 50266

All Scripture quotations, unless otherwise noted, are from the Holy Bible, New International Version © 2011 Biblica, Inc.

First Edition, 2018

Library of Congress Control Number: 2017950799

Author Academy Elite, Powell, Ohio

Printed in the United States of America

Paperback: 978-1-64085-093-4
Hardback: 978-1-64085-204-4
Ebook: 978-1-64085-094-1

DEDICATION

To the growing number of wellness and medical professionals who are working to create a new healthcare system based on preventing disease.

CONTENTS

ACKNOWLEDGMENTS

The mentoring of the John Maxwell Team helped me establish practices that improved the writing process and content. Author Academy Elite provided a process that helped create a much improved final product.

Dr. Joe Figueroa provided very valuable insights on the practical aspects of effective interactions with patients.

Fiverr editors vastly reduced the amount of time spent on areas like references, proofreading and grammar.

Jetlaunch did a great job on the cover.

INTRODUCTION

The Great American Low-Fat Diet Experiment

I lived in England for three years in the late nineties (1990s). The cultural differences immediately stood out when I first arrived. Everything seemed different in some way from America, including routine activities. Some differences were large and others small. One of the first things that I noticed at the grocery store was the lack of low-fat foods which had become an established craze in America. Even more surprising, the British populace was obviously thinner than America's population in spite of the lack of low-fat foods. At the time, I was convinced of the low-fat dogma, so I really didn't know what to make of the observation. It couldn't be that low-fat, high-carb was unhealthy. In fact, I worried that I would become unhealthy if I didn't find some low-fat foods soon!

This was the same period when medical and health professionals were becoming aware of the extent of the diabetes and obesity epidemics in America. Up to this time, most health professionals also believed the low-fat dogma because of the poor quality and quantity of nutrition research. Little did we know that healthy dietary fat does not translate to fat on our bodies.

The contribution of the low-fat/high-carb dogma to America's obesity problem is no longer a mystery. There has been a 40-year war between brain and body in America, and the weapons of warfare have been low-fat, high-carb, and highly processed foods. The data is before us (1):

- About 70% of our population is overweight or obese

- There are more obese people than overweight people

- Extreme obesity is growing the fastest

- The majority of overweight people have been following a low-fat, high-carb diet for decades

The biggest increase in obesity rates occurred between the late 1970s and the late 1990s (1). Scientists went to work to figure out what low-fat, high-carb diets do and they have answers. Low-fat, high-carb diets trigger the hoarding of calories by the fat cells (2). We've been fighting against the natural design of our own metabolism. It's not primarily a lack of willpower. The bullet points above can be thought of as an unofficial, nationwide study with the largest possible sample size. In a sense, we did the study by experimenting on ourselves.

Companies that thrive on low-fat, high-carb, highly processed foods will continue to portray low-fat, high-carb diets as healthy. However, more people are recognizing the impact of a high-carbohydrate diet. Soft drink sales have been declining for over 10 years (3). Coke and Pepsi appear to be recognizing these trends. As a result, they are bringing more healthy drinks to the market. By 2017, bottled water is likely to surpass soft drink sales (3). Producers of highly processed foods would do well to recognize these trends and reorient themselves around healthy products.

1. National Institute of Diabetes and Digestive and Kidney Diseases. (2012). Overweight & obesity statistics. Retrieved from https://www.niddk.nih.gov/health-information/health-statistics/Pages/overweight-obesity-statistics.aspx

2. Ludwig, D. (2016). Always hungry: Conquer cravings, retrain your fat cells, and lose weight permanently. New York, NY: Grand Central Publishing.

3. Esterl, M. (2015, March). Soft drinks hit 10th year of decline: Diet soda volumes fall sharply, bottled water makes gains. The Wall Street Journal. Retrieved from http://www.wsj.com/articles/pepsi-cola-replaces-diet-coke-as-no-2-soda-1427388559

The impact of soft drinks and convenience foods on children

Type 2 diabetes did not impact young people historically. The first type 2 diabetes cases in children occurred in recent history (1,2,3,4,5,6). The increase in type 2 diabetes (T2D) correlates with the rise in convenience foods and the placement of pop machines in schools. Childhood diabetes is no longer overwhelmingly type 1. Historically, type 1 was referred to as childhood onset, and type 2 was referred to as adult onset. With the rise in convenience foods and soft drinks, childhood T2D began to increase to the point that it almost exceeds the level of type 1 diabetes in some locations. Childhood type 2 diabetes is particularly important because it clarifies that behavior patterns can have major impacts at an early age. "It is estimated that type 2 diabetes mellitus (T2D) represents 8–45% of patients with diabetes mellitus currently diagnosed in large US pediatric centers; however, this is likely to be an underestimation and incidence is probably rising" (4). "In the UK, hospital admissions in type 2 diabetic patients below 18 years of age rose by approximately 45% between 1996–97 and

2003–04. This parallels the 63% rise in patient admission for obesity in the same period. In the US, diabetes-related hospitalization rate has increased by ~40% between 1993–2004 among those aged 20–29 years" (5). A 45% increase nationally in 7 years is very significant. In spite of this evidence, many people are still resistant to accepting the behavioral basis of type 2 diabetes. Some of the clearest statistics that impact a person's awareness of the behavioral basis of type 2 diabetes include:

- Childhood type 2 diabetes did not exist at any significant level before the rise in convenience foods

- 33% of people born today will have type 2 diabetes within their lifetime (8)

- The impact of sugar on type 2 diabetes has the same trend with different ethnic compositions, indicating that this trend does not depend on culture or race (7)

T2D is a behavioral disease. A behavioral approach is needed to prevent or reverse it. Lifestyle factors are driving the rise in obesity and insulin resistance. According to a study by Song and Hardisty (7), soft drinks consumption has substantially increased, and clinical studies have linked this to the rise in obesity and type 2 diabetes in children, adolescents, and young adults. The Bogal USA Heart Study demonstrated an association between consumption of sweetened soft drinks and metabolic syndrome in young adults (9). Soft drink consumption is an indicator of other behaviors associated with type 2 diabetes such as a greater intake of calories and saturated and trans fat, lower consumption of fiber and dairy products, and sedentary lifestyle.

1. D'Adamo, E., & Caprio, S. (2011). Type 2 diabetes in youth: Epidemiology and pathophysiology. Diabetes

Care, 34(Suppl 2), S161-S165. https://doi.org/10.2337/dc11-s212

2. Taubes, G. (2016). The case against sugar. New York, NY: Alfred A. Knopf Publisher.

3. Pulgaron, E. R., & Delamater, A. M. (2014). Obesity and type 2 diabetes in children: Epidemiology and treatment. Current Diabetes Reports, 14(8), 508. doi:10.1007/s11892-014-0508-y

4. Reinehr, T. (2013). Type 2 diabetes mellitus in children and adolescents. World Journal of Diabetes, 4(6), 270-281. doi:10.4239/wjd.v4.i6.270

5. Dyer, O. (2002). First cases of type 2 diabetes found in white UK teenagers. BMJ, 324(7336), 506.

6. Fagot-Campagna, A. (2000). Emergence of type 2 diabetes mellitus in children: Epidemiological evidence. Journal of Pediatric Endocrinology and Metabolism, 13(Suppl 6), 1395-1402.

7. Song, S. H., & Hardisty, C. A. (2008). Early-onset type 2 diabetes mellitus: An increasing phenomenon of elevated cardiovascular risk. Medscape, 6(3), 315-322.

8. Boyle, J. P. et al. (2010). Projection of the year 2050 burden of diabetes in the US adult population: dynamic modeling of incidence, mortality, and prediabetes prevalence. *Popul Health Metr.,*8(29), 1-12. doi:10.1186/1478-7954-8-29

9. Freedman, D. S. (1999). The Relation of Overweight to Cardiovascular Risk Factors Among Children and Adolescents: The Bogalusa Heart Study. Pediatrics,103(6).

The epidemics of chronic disease

Did you know that type 2 diabetes is 100% preventable and highly reversible (1)? If a person were to eat a healthy diet their entire life, maintain a healthy weight, and exercise regularly, they would not acquire type 2 diabetes. Even when people have had it many years, much of the damage can be reversed. The longer a person has had type 2 diabetes, the lower the chances of reversal. Nonetheless, anyone at any stage can initiate positive change that can occur by making the switch to a healthy lifestyle and maintaining it. We can naturally control the speed with which sugar enters into our bodies. If we minimize the intake of sugar and moderate the speed of uptake, it helps balance our blood sugar maintenance needs. Healthy living also helps our pocketbook. The degree to which prevention takes precedence over treatment determines our prescription bills and impacts our quality of life.

T2D is one of the major chronic diseases that affect almost every American family and increasingly the rest of the world. Infectious disease is still largely under the control of the tools of modern medicine. Not so for chronic disease because they are mostly behavioral conditions. Heart disease, diabetes, stroke, and cancer are all driven by poor diet, insufficient exercise, tobacco use, and stress. All of these factors are behavioral and account for approximately 84% of chronic disease healthcare costs. If we can prevent or, in many cases, reverse chronic disease, why are more Americans not getting healthy?

There are many factors that contribute to health status. Behavior-driven chronic diseases are dependent on our choices and our environment. Most chronic disease would not exist if people maintained a healthy lifestyle. Rates of chronic disease are very low in indigenous populations unaffected by the Western diet (3). Our choices are within our control. Our environment is almost entirely outside our control. Seven different areas are within our ability to modify for the better, including spiritual health, relational health, mental health, emotional health, physical health, vocational health, and financial health. If we don't take positive control of these areas, each of them will ultimately impact our physical health. That was my story. I was unhealthy in every area of non-physical health, and it affected my physical health in major ways. At one point, both my HDL and LDL categories were officially classified as "high risk."

Non-physical health issues reinforce poor eating and exercise habits. Comfort eating is one of the most common ways to cope with stress. Comfort eating easily becomes addictive because addictive foods are available at home, work, convenience stores, and shopping centers. Even well-meaning family and friends offer us addictive food on a regular basis. Addictive food contains high levels of sugar, flour, salt, fat, and processed ingredients. High sugar processed foods are clinically measurable as addictive agents according to the Yale food addiction scale (4).

The impact of sugar on food addiction plays a major role in the diabetes epidemic. Food and sugar addiction drive the eating habits that lead to insulin resistance and T2D development. Sugar is so impactful that it can be singled out from all other factors. A Stanford study showed that sugar was strongly correlated with the onset of type 2 diabetes independent of other factors such as ethnicity, sedentary behavior, and other food types. In fact, differences in sugar availability "statistically explain variations in diabetes prevalence rates" (5). Few studies have this level of clarity and mutually reinforcing data across a broad spectrum of over 100 nations.

1. Hyman, M. (2012). The blood sugar solution: The ultrahealthy program for losing weight, preventing disease, and feeling great now!. New York, NY: Little, Brown and Company.

2. *Moses H 3rd, Matheson DH, Dorsey ER, George BP, Sadoff D, Yoshimura S JAMA. 2013 Nov 13; 310(18):1947-63.* doi: 10.1001/jama.2013.281425

3. Taubes, G. (2016). The case against sugar. New York, NY: Alfred A. Knopf Publisher.

4. Fast Lab. (n.d.). Food and addiction science & treatment lab. Retrieved from http://fastlab.psych.lsa.umich.edu/yale-food-addiction-scale/

5. Basu, S., Yoffe, P., Hills, N., & Lustig, R. H. (2013). The relationship of sugar to population-level diabetes prevalence: An econometric analysis of repeated cross-sectional data. PLoS One, 8(2), e57873.

5 out of 7 billion people lack a healthy diet

Diet makes a major contribution to each of the major chronic diseases mentioned. According to The World Food Center (WFC) at UC Davis, there are 1.9 billion adults who are overweight or obese, 795 million who are underweight, and 2 billion who may consume enough calories but lack the necessary micronutrients (1). The WFC has identified nutrition as a multidimensional problem and providing a healthy global diet will require:

- Interdisciplinary science
- Food supply
- Food safety
- Clean water
- Sanitation
- Poverty alleviation
- Education
- Health care access

A Nielsen study helps us understand the availability of healthy food in various parts of the world and the impact of social norms on diet quality (2).

- Asia Pacific: "Consumers in Asia Pacific lead the world when it comes to intention to purchase organics (47% compared to global average of 40%). Compared to the global average, Asia Pacific consumers who actively buy organics are most likely to do so because they view organics as healthier (82% vs. global average of 76%) and more nutritious (57% vs. 51%)."

- Europe: Important diet considerations included: locally-made products, distance from point-of-origin, limited product packaging, and no animal testing all rated high on the scale of factors that were important when shopping.

- North America: Expense was the primary reason Americans do not eat healthy, along with an unwillingness to sacrifice taste. Environmental and social considerations drive the purchasing of organics, making it the region most likely to "buy organics to avoid toxins (71%), promote environmentally-friendly organic farms (59%), help small farmers (58%), avoid genetically-modified products (45%), do the right thing (38%) and vote against modern farming methods (23%)."

- Middle East/Africa/Pakistan: Time and expense associated with healthy eating pose the lowest barriers to this region in which consumers find a scarcity of healthy eating options (31%) and are confused as to which foods are really healthy (30%). This region is most likely (29%) to select products that come from farmer's markets.

The consumption of white rice as a staple is contributing strongly to the rise of T2D in Asia. Eating white rice and refined grains is associated with increased risk of developing type 2 diabetes (3). Harvard School of Public Health researchers from the Department of Nutrition reviewed four studies involving more than 352,000 people from China, Japan, the United States, and Australia who were tracked between four and 22 years. Those who ate the most rice—three to four servings a day—were 1.5 times more likely to have diabetes than people who ate the least amount of rice. In addition, "for every additional large bowl of white rice a person ate each day, the risk rose 10 percent. The link was stronger for people in Asian countries, who eat an average of three to four servings of white rice per day. People in Western countries eat, on average, one to two servings a week" (4). White rice has a high glycemic index leading to spikes in blood sugar.

1. World Food Center. (n.d.). Building healthier outcomes from our food system. Retrieved from http://worldfoodcenter.ucdavis.edu/About/nutrition.html

2. Newswire. (n.d.). Global trends in healthy eating. Retrieved from http://www.nielsen.com/us/en/insights/news/2010/global-trends-in-healthy-eating.html

3. Asian Diabetes Prevention Initiative. (n.d.). Why are Asians at higher risk?. Retrieved from http://asiandiabetesprevention.org/what-is-diabetes/why-are-asians-higher-risk

4. Hu, E. A., Pan, A., Malik, V., & Sun, Q. (2012). White rice consumption and risk of type 2 diabetes: Meta-analysis and systematic review. BMJ, 344, e1454. https://doi.org/10.1136/bmj.e1454

Chronic disease accounts for half of all deaths

According to the CDC, chronic diseases are the leading causes of death and disability in the United States. These include heart disease, stroke, cancer, type 2 diabetes, obesity, and arthritis. These are among the most common, costly, and preventable of all health problems. More than half of the population has a chronic disease. 50% of the American adult population has either prediabetes or diabetes (1). Many adults have more than one chronic disease. The CDC estimates that one of four adults had two or more chronic health conditions (2).

Seven of the top 10 causes of death in 2010 were chronic diseases (3). Heart disease and cancer together accounted for nearly 48% of all deaths (2). Infectious disease has been replaced by chronic disease as the leading cause of death throughout the developed world. The good news is that most chronic diseases are preventable. Type 2 diabetes is the most preventable. It does not occur if a healthy diet is maintained. Diabetes is linked through diet to the top 2 causes of death, heart disease, and cancer.

Number of deaths for leading causes of death according to the CDC (5):

- Heart disease: 614,348
- Cancer: 591,699
- Chronic lower respiratory diseases: 147,101
- Accidents (unintentional injuries): 136,053
- Stroke (cerebrovascular diseases): 133,103
- Alzheimer's disease: 93,541
- Diabetes: 76,488

- Influenza and Pneumonia: 55,227
- Nephritis, nephrotic syndrome, and nephrosis: 48,146
- Intentional self-harm (suicide): 42,773

More than 1 million Americans and more than 10 million people worldwide are expected to be diagnosed with cancer this year (4). America's population is only 4% of the global population, but it has 10% of the cancer cases. This suggests that environment and lifestyle contribute to cancer onset in the U.S. For example, cancer is a genetic disease in the sense that mutations generate cancer. However, only a small percent of cancers are due to inherited genetic defects. Most cancerous genetic defects are preventable.

1. Menke, A., Casagrande, S., Geiss, L., & Cowie, C. C. (2015). Prevalence of and trends in diabetes among adults in the United States. *JAMA, 314*(10), 1021-1029. doi:10.1001/jama.2015.10029

2. Centers for Disease Control and Prevention. (2016). Chronic disease prevention and health promotion. Retrieved from https://www.cdc.gov/chronicdisease/resources/publications/aag/diabetes.htm

3. Centers for Disease Control and Prevention. (2017). Deaths and mortality. *National Center for Health Statistics*. Retrieved from http://www.cdc.gov/nchs/fastats/deaths.htm

4. Anand, P., Kunnumakara, A. B., Sundaram, C., Harikumar, K. B., Tharakan, S. T., Lai, O. S., ..., & Aggarwar, B. B. (2008). Cancer is a preventable disease that requires major lifestyle changes. Pharmaceutical Research, 25(9), 2097-2116. doi:10.1007/s11095-008-9661-9

5. Centers for Disease Control and Prevention. (2017). Deaths and mortality. *National Center for Health Statistics*. Retrieved from http://www.cdc.gov/nchs/fastats/deaths.htm

Chronic disease is a global but solvable problem

Chronic disease is not only the leading cause of death in the United States, but it was also responsible for 5 of the 10 leading causes of death worldwide in 2015, including the top two. In 2000, only two of the top 10 were major chronic diseases (heart disease and stroke) (1). Diabetes was not in the top 10 in 2000, but it moved to number 6 by 2015 (1). The current transition to global diet-driven disease is occurring rapidly. Most disease problems in the world today are chronic diseases such as obesity, diabetes, heart disease, and cancer. This is a historical trend. Before the development of large-scale vaccination programs and antibiotics, infectious disease generated the most serious health problems and epidemics. Infectious disease is largely under control in developed nations because of developments in vaccinations and medications. Now the most significant health issues in developed nations are epidemics of chronic disease due to diet and lifestyle.

Although lifestyle based disease is still a difficult problem, it is an easier problem to solve scientifically than infectious disease. Scientists and community leaders were unaware of the root causes of infectious disease before the discovery of bacteria and viruses and the means of preventing their infection. Today, we have the major advantage of knowing the lifestyle root causes of most major chronic diseases. Successful lifestyle change programs are currently in existence, and these programs can lead the way forward for addressing chronic disease.

1. World Health Organization. (2017).
    The top 10 causes of death. Retrieved from
    http://www.who.int/mediacentre/factsheets/fs310/en/

PART 1
THE RELATIONSHIP BETWEEN DIET AND CHRONIC DISEASE

1
HISTORICAL DEVELOPMENT OF CHRONIC DISEASE EPIDEMICS

How did an addictive food environment develop globally?

THE ARRIVAL OF the low-fat, high-carb craze began in the 1970s when fat was demonized. This was based on studies that considered only the caloric content of food and not the chemical structure and how it interacts with biological organisms. Fat has the highest number of calories per gram of the major food groups, and it became the scapegoat of chronic disease—especially heart disease. In many ways, the low-fat, high-carb craze initiated a journey of pain for many Americans and people throughout the world. It has been manifested in the following ways:

- The pain of obesity
- The pain of the difficulty of weight loss (made much harder by a low-fat diet that works against human metabolism)

- The pain of chronic disease
- The pain of carb crashes and cravings
- The pain of always being hungry

Availability of simple carbohydrates is a key factor in consumption levels. Sugar became available in America in the early sixteen-hundreds (1). The lack of sugar availability kept early consumption levels of sugar low. Early sugar consumption levels were estimated to be about 20 teaspoons of sugar per person per year (2).

> The average American consumes 77–150 pounds of added sugar annually. Americans consume an additional 150 pounds per year of flour

Historic levels of sugar consumption in England began at about 4 pounds per person per year in 1700. By 1900, consumption increased to 100 pounds a year, a 25-fold increase. Similar trends have occurred worldwide with the increasing availability of convenience foods, fast food, snacks, and sugary drinks. Sugar consumption was given a further push by the low-fat craze. As fat was taken out of food, sugar was added in to improve flavor.

Historic levels of sugar consumption (3)

- In 1700, the average Englishman consumed 4 pounds a year
- 1800: the average man ate 18 pounds of sugar (4.5-fold increase)
- 1870: 47 pounds annually (10 fold)
- 1900: up to 100 pounds a year (25 fold)

- Today: The average American consumes 77–150 pounds of added sugar annually. Americans consume an additional 150 pounds per year of flour (4)

Even though our food environment has changed dramatically, it was a gradual change. Over several decades, we became a nation saturated in addictive foods. Addictive foods are highly processed foods containing flour, sugar, salt, and fat (5,6). Iowa State University Extension has a newsletter called Words on Wellness. Recently, they published an article on processed foods. Processed foods make up about 60% of the calories in products from the grocery store. It appears that over half of the American diet on average is made of processed foods.

1. Sugar in Early American History. (2011, September 7). Retrieved from http://www.alcademics.com/2011/09/sugar-in-early-american-history.html

2. Hyman, M. (2013, November 12). Why You Should Never Eat High Fructose Corn Syrup. Retrieved from http://www.huffingtonpost.com/dr-mark-hyman/high-fructose-corn-syrup_b_4256220.html

3. Cohen, R. (2013, August). Sugar Love. Retrieved from http://ngm.nationalgeographic.com/2013/08/sugar/cohen-text

4. Hyman, M. (2016). *Eat fat, get thin: why the fat we eat is the key to sustained weight loss and vibrant health*. New York: Little, Brown and Company.

5. Food and Addiction Science & Treatment Lab. (n.d.). Retrieved May 26, 2017, from http://fastlab.psych.lsa.umich.edu/yale-food-addiction-scale/

6. 9 Charts That Show Why America is Fat, Sick & Tired. (n.d.). Retrieved May 26, 2017, from https://draxe.com/charts-american-diet/

What led to all the processed foods? The low-fat craze which began in the 1970s. Nutrition guidelines recommended low-fat, high-carb diets. The food industry jumped on board and created supermarkets full of granola bars, bagels, donuts, low-fat cookies, whole grain cereals, and a multitude of other snacks. The combination of government nutrition guidelines and the ubiquitous supply of low-fat foods claiming to be healthy convinced most people that low-fat foods are healthy.

A research article by Popkin et al. describes how diets in the 1970s in America began to shift toward an increased reliance upon (1):

- processed foods
- restaurant food
- unhealthy edible oils
- sugar-sweetened beverages

The typical American diet consists of about 50% carbohydrate, 15% protein, and 35% fat (2). Reduced physical activity and increased sedentary time coincided with these diet changes. These changes began in the low- and middle-income countries in the early 1990s but did not become clearly recognized until diabetes, hypertension, and obesity began to dominate the globe. Both the poorest and higher income countries experienced rapid increases in overweight and obesity status. These trends were accompanied by concurrent rapid shifts in diet and activity. Despite the major health challenges faced, few countries are adequately addressing the dietary challenges generated by processed food.

American and many other nations are consuming unusually high levels of sugar, and other addictive substances in our food ... much higher levels than our bodies can handle, as evidenced by the emergence of diet-driven diseases, including diabetes, heart disease, cancer, and Alzheimer's. Chronic disease has spread wherever the western diet has been introduced. High-sugar, low-fat snacks are full of highly processed ingredients that actually program our fat cells to hoard calories. This occurs because carbohydrates are the most stimulatory food for insulin production. Insulin then triggers the fat cells to take up calories from the blood. Unfortunately, the brain only senses the low glucose in the blood and not the calories in the fat cells. Therefore, our brain thinks we're starving when actually all the calories are hidden in the fat cells.

Total consumption of simple carbohydrates per person is estimated to be 300 pounds per year (3). This is more than a 70-fold increase in the annual intake of simple carbohydrates since the 1700s. At this level of historical increase, it would be surprising if these consumption rates did not result in adverse consequences. 300 pounds of simple carbs per year is equivalent to almost 10 Cokes per day (39 g sugar/ 12 oz Coke). Much of this comes in the form of bread, rice, pasta, and cereal instead of Coke. This level of consumption is toxic to our bodies. It tests the limit of what our bodies can handle. The historical trends give us clues as to what level of sugar consumption is safe. It appears that type 2 diabetes did not appear historically in the common population until sugar consumption increased above approximately 20 pounds per person per year (4). One 12 oz can of Coke per day provides about three times that amount. The historical record indicates that the diabetes epidemic did not begin until the 19th century when sugar consumption rose from 18 pounds per person per year in 1800 to 100 pounds per year by 1900. Somewhere within the range between 20 and 100 pounds of sugar consumption per year are quantities where sugar consumption is high enough to initiate chronic disease. It appears that the highest diabetes rates which occurred in the late 1990s until around 2013 required even higher levels of sugar consumption. Further scientific studies can probably relate diabetes onset to more exact levels of sugar consumption.

1. Popkin, B. M., Adair, L., & Ng, S. (2013). NOW AND THEN: The Global Nutrition Transition: The Pandemic of Obesity in Developing Countries. *Nutr Rev.,70* (1), 3-21.

2. Last, L. R., & Wilson, S. A. (2006). Low-Carbohydrate Diets. *American Family Physician,73*(11), 1942-1948.

3. Hyman, M. (2016). *Eat fat, get thin: why the fat we eat is the key to sustained weight loss and vibrant health.* New York: Little, Brown and Company. p.13.

4. Taubes, G. (2017). *The case against sugar.* New York: Alfred A. Knopf.

Historical trends in diabetes and the food environment

Healthy eating became much more challenging during and after the advent of the Great Prosperity following World War 2. The unprecedented increase in wealth in the United States led to faster lifestyles requiring fast food. Fast food and comfort food became increasingly available during this period. The rise in type 2 diabetes prevalence correlates with sugar consumption demographically and historically. As the consumption of sugar processed foods and sugary drinks has increased, so has the rate of type 2 diabetes (1). The beginning of the first linear phase T2D epidemic was in the late 1950s (2). A second linear phase with a steeper slope began in the mid-1990s.

Total Pre-Diabetic and Diabetic Population
Pre-diabetes or diabetes: About 50% of American adults (3)
Diabetes: 9.3% (29.1 million Americans) (4)

Type 2 diabetes emerges in populations in approximately 12–20 years after the introduction of a Western-style diet (5). It took 40–50 years for diabetes and diet-driven disease to have high enough health impacts in the U.S. for people to take notice and act. Because it took so long to understand the drivers of chronic disease, most people, including doctors, didn't think it was a problem. Another important factor was the asymptomatic nature of pre-diabetes and early-stage diabetes. By the time symptoms arrive, type 2 diabetes is much harder to reverse.

> Type 2 diabetes emerges in populations approximately 12–20 years after the introduction of a Western-style diet

1. Basu, S. et al. (2013). The Relationship of Sugar to Population-Level Diabetes Prevalence: An Econometric Analysis of Repeated Cross-Sectional Data. *PLOS one,8*(2), 1-8. doi:10.1371/journal.pone.0057873

2. Long-term Trends in Diabetes . (2017, April). Retrieved from https://www.cdc.gov/diabetes/statistics/slides/long_term_trends.pdf

3. Menke, A. et al. (2015). Prevalence of and Trends in Diabetes Among Adults in the United States. *JAMA,314*(10), 1021-1029. doi:doi:10.1001/jama.2015.10029

4. Statistics about Diabetes. (2014, June 10). American Diabetes Association. Retrieved 2015, from http://www.diabetes.org/diabetes-basics/statistics/

5. Taubes, G. (2017). *The case against sugar*. New York: Alfred A. Knopf, Ch 2

The availability of convenience foods impacts health

American fast food began in the early 1900s with White Castle and A & W restaurants and picked up speed in the post-World War 2 economic boom,1945–1975. Spending on fast food has increased from $6 billion in 1970 to $110 billion in 2000, an 18-fold increase. Americans spend more money on fast food than on higher education, personal computers, computer software, or new cars (1). The top 15 fast food chains in the nation have 105,000 total stores which saturate the landscape (2).

Consider the following list of businesses where high-sugar food and drinks are marketed aggressively (3,4):

- Convenience Stores 2016   154,195
- Drugstores   41,969
- Superettes/Supermarkets/Supercenter   51,055
- Dollar Stores   27,378
- Restaurants over 600,000 in the U.S.

Convenience stores grew with the development of interstate systems, urbanization, and the push for faster service and faster food. They are located in the highest traffic areas and are the closest stores to interstate exits. As a result, they have become favorite stopping points for travelers. These stores sell addictive, processed foods, and high-sugar drinks. The entire back wall of most convenience stores consists of sweetened drinks and processed foods. Candy and processed foods make up much of the remaining shelf space. Thus, one-third to two-thirds of the retail space in a convenience store is occupied by high-sugar foods and drinks. Our food environment saturates us in high-carb, processed foods almost everywhere we go. A study by Fuzhong et al. found a significant association between increased density of neighborhood fast-food outlets with "unhealthy lifestyles, poorer psychosocial profiles, and increased risk of obesity among older adults" (5).

Washington, Illinois is a small town of 15,000 about 7 miles south of where I grew up. It is a good example of the daily exposure to processed foods and high-sugar drinks. Most people use business Route 24 to commute to work in town or the surrounding area. Most commuters pass between 15 and 25 locations where processed foods and high-sugar drinks are the most popular items. This high-level availability combined with the carb craving cycle almost precludes a healthy diet for most Americans who lack awareness of how these foods affect our bodies. This high availability of convenience foods is a dominant factor leading to their consumption. Eating carbs stimulates cravings more than eating fat or protein. Carbs also stimulate repeat craving cycles (6). In the current food environment, people accept inadequate self-care because it's the cultural norm of a high-carb, low-fat, fast food society. Awareness is building of how dangerous this cultural norm is to our health and how we can engage in healthy alternatives. Healthy non-deprivation diets that taste great and help people feel full are becoming more common.

Convenience food trends became established over approximately four decades. During that time, a large infrastructure has been put in place that supports the continuation of current increases in obesity and T2D. The infrastructure of convenience stores and fast food restaurants makes changing trends more difficult. However, the current infrastructure does not need to be disassembled in order to address obesity trends. Many fast food restaurants have begun to feature healthy alternatives. Because healthy food is at least as delicious as unhealthy food, it is possible that new restaurant chains could take advantage of the market opportunity to offer delicious, healthy fast food. Success by such restaurants could then stimulate change in existing restaurant chains. Alternatively, many existing chains may decide to pursue the healthy food market opportunities.

I struggled with carb cravings and carb crashes for decades. My breakfast was dominated by carbohydrates on a daily basis. I thought I was eating a healthy breakfast because I was following the government's food pyramid. Around mid-morning and mid-afternoon, my mind almost ceased to function because it was so overwhelmed by brain fog. Paying attention in lectures or meetings was almost impossible because I was unable to concentrate or think. My diet consisted almost entirely of carbohydrates: Breakfast consisted of bagels, cereal, or fruit every day. Lunch was almost always some type of pasta. Supper was often cereal or pasta. If I went out to eat at a restaurant, I ate several slices of bread thinking that it was healthy. Many days, I ate almost 100% carbs (cereal for breakfast and supper; pasta for lunch).

What about high-carb foods in the workplace? Large organizations employ about half of the workforce. Based on the size of the employer, 50–80% of the workforce is exposed to vending machines in the workplace (7). The total businesses that expose their employees to high-sugar foods at socials or meetings is probably close to 100%. This means that daily exposure to unhealthy, high-sugar foods is highly probable for most of the workforce.

Another established norm that inhibits the transition to a healthier food environment is the preference for treatment over prevention. Many would rather take medication than change lifestyle patterns. Advanced medicine has allowed people to make this choice. In spite of the epidemic rise and type 2 diabetes, heart disease and cancer, survival rates have increased significantly because of the advancements in medical technology and pharmaceuticals. If survival rates are improving and lifespans are long, most people do not sense an immediate need to change the treatment paradigms in health care. However, treatment is far inferior to prevention in terms of long-term health care costs individually or collectively. Treatment also decreases the quality of life and enables food addiction cycles.

1. Schlosser, E. (2007). *Fast food nation*. Barcelona: Debolsillo.

2. McConnell, A., & Bhasin, K. (2012, June 12). RANKED: The Most Popular Fast Food Restaurants In America. Retrieved from http://www.businessinsider.com/the-most-popular-fast-food-restaurants-in-america-2012-7

3. U.S. Convenience Store Count (2017) Retrieved from http://www.nacsonline.com/research/factsheets/scopeofindustry/pages/industrystorecount.aspx

4. U.S. Total Restaurant Count Increases by 4,442 Units over Last Year, Reports NPD. (2013, January 23). Retrieved from https://www.npd.com/wps/portal/npd/us/news/press-releases/us-total-restaurant-count-increases-by-4442-units-over-last-year-reports-npd/

5. Li, F. et al. (2009). Obesity and the Built Environment: Does the Density of Neighborhood Fast-Food Outlets Matter? *Am J Health Promot., 23*(3), 203-209. doi:10.4278/ajhp.071214133

6. Ludwig, D. (2016). *Always Hungry*. New York, NY: Grand Central Life and Style., p. 61

7. Caruso, A. (2015, February). Statistics of U.S. Businesses Employment and Payroll Summary: 2012. Retrieved from https://www.census.gov/content/dam/Census/library/publications/2015/econ/g12-susb.pdf

Trends in obesity

The diabetes trends described above are closely related to obesity. However, obesity does not cause diabetes. Instead, they are diet-driven diseases that reinforce each other. Trends in obesity have paralleled the trends in type 2 diabetes and the food environment. The same foods that drive diabetes onset also drive weight gain. This creates the advantage of reversing multiple conditions simultaneously simply by making the change to a healthy diet. The obesity summary charts clarify the time periods in which obesity, diabetes, and changes in the food environment occurred simultaneously.

Historical rate of rise in obesity and T2D
100% Increase in obesity from late 1970s to 2007–2008 (1)
The prevalence of obesity increased from 21% in 1997 to 29% in 2006 (2)
"88% of all Americans don't get enough exercise." — Mark Hyman, MD

1. Finkelstein, E. A. (2012). Obesity and Severe Obesity Forecasts Through 2030. *Am J Prev Med,42*(6), 563-570.

2. Alley, D. et al. (2012) Changes in the Association Between Body Mass Index and Medicare Costs, 1997–2006.. *Arch Intern Med,172*(3), 277-278. doi:doi:10.1001/archinternmed.2011.702

Total Overweight or Obese Population Overweight & Obesity Statistics. (n.d.). Retrieved May 27, 2017, from https://www.niddk.nih.gov/health-information/health-statistics/overweight-obesity
Total percent overweight (adult): 69%
Child and adolescent obesity: 34%

Trends in extreme obesity
Extreme obesity was very rare before the early 1970s (1)
Extreme obesity has increased faster than obesity (2)

1. Finkelstein, E. A. (2012). Obesity and Severe Obesity Forecasts Through 2030. *Am J Prev Med,42*(6), 563-570. Retrieved May 27, 2017, from http://www.ajpmonline.org/article/S0749-3797(12)00146-8/pdf

2. Overweight & Obesity Statistics. (n.d.). Retrieved May 27, 2017, from https://www.niddk.nih.gov/health-information/health-statistics/overweight-obesity

Economic impact of chronic disease

The US ranks 43 in health and wellness

Trends in diet-driven disease have impacted the U.S. economically. The World Economic Forum generates an annual report called Human Capital. The Human Capital report is based on measuring 4 different pillars of human productivity. The ranking of the United States for each of the categories is listed below out of 122 countries (1):

Workforce and employment: 4
Education: 11
Enabling environment: 16
Health and wellness: 43

1. The Human Capital Report. (n.d.). Retrieved May 27, 2017, from http://www3.weforum.org/docs/WEF_HumanCapitalReport_2013.pdf

The US's greatest strength is threatened by its greatest weakness

The US's greatest strength is threatened by its greatest weakness. In the Human Capital Index (HCI), the US's highest rank among the HCI pillars is in workforce and employment. However, its lowest ranking is health and wellness. America's ranking for the business impact of non-communicable (chronic) disease is 112 out of 122 (1). Thus, chronic disease gives the US one of the lowest rankings out of any country in this business impact category.

> America's ranking for the business impact of non-communicable (chronic) disease is 112 out of 122

The impact of chronic disease on business can eventually impact the economy in significant ways. These HCI rankings point the way towards a solution. Since chronic illness is the biggest threat to the business community, investing in health and wellness could be the best way to invest in business, the economy, and our communities. The path toward implementing wellness in the workplace and elsewhere is known. Effective programs are widely available but not yet widely used.

The U.S. ranked in the lower half of countries for obesity, stress, depression, and business impact of chronic disease. Here is the U.S. ranking among 122 countries in several wellness categories:

Healthcare quality 29
Life expectancy 30
Unhealthy life years (% of life expectancy) 34
Healthcare accessibility 50
Depression (% of respondents) 65
Stress (% of respondents) 106
Obesity (% of adults with BMI ≥ 30) 112
Business impact of non-communicable diseases 112

1. The Human Capital Report. (n.d.). Retrieved May 27, 2017, from http://www3.weforum.org/docs/WEF_HumanCapitalReport_2013.pdf

America's health status and why we can't stay here

The current and projected levels of chronic disease from obesity and diabesity is not sustainable personally, financially, or communally. Two-thirds of our population is overweight or obese. If we remain in present patterns of food consumption, scientists and medical professionals are increasingly concerned that the future burden will overwhelm our health care system's finances and personnel resources. The projected 33% T2D rate by 2050 is intrinsically linked with other diet-driven diseases (cancer, obesity, heart disease, Alzheimer's). The cost of this level of T2D alone is problematic for the economy and our communities. Combine T2D with the costs of the other major chronic diseases and the total cost is unsustainable. Dr. Mike Roizen, Cleveland Clinic wellness director, estimates that a doubling of tax rates may be needed by 2025 to cover the cost of chronic health care (1).

1. How healthcare impacts community sustainability [Interview by T. Schierer]. (2016, December 28). Interview with Dr. Mike Roizen at the Cleveland Clinic

CDC estimate for T2D diagnosis: 33% by 2050 (1)

Sugar has the capability to drive diabetes rate increases in the absence of obesity and several other factors. As a Stanford study clearly demonstrated, over a hundred foreign countries experienced significant diabetes increases independent of obesity (2). Even with a successful reduction of obesity, diabetes trends could continue because of the independent impact of sugar.

Cost of T2D
Total medical costs per person with T2D: Twice the cost of someone without T2D (2.3x; 3)
National Cost: $245 billion (2013); this is the total cost of diabetes and includes medical costs, lost work, and lost wages (3)

Cost Increases in Obesity and T2D
2007: $174 billion; 7.6% (4)
2013: $245 billion; 8.4% (4)
2030: $861 to 957 billion; 16–18% (5)

Spending increases on health conditions related to obesity (6)
Obesity-attributable spending increase for diabetes: 38 percent
Obesity-attributable spending increase for hyperlipidemia: 22 percent
Obesity-attributable spending increase for heart disease: 41 percent

Untreated chronic disease results in high end of life health-care costs for individuals and a substantial portion of overall health care costs. A recent analysis of U.S. health care spending revealed that chronic illnesses account for 84% of total health care costs (7). According to the movie Fed Up, 95% of Americans will be overweight by 2050 (8). Currently, 40% of non-obese people are metabolically obese. The Brookings Institute found that lifetime societal costs were $92,235 greater for a person with obesity ($2013), at a 3 percent discount rate. Using this estimate, if all 12.7 million U.S. youth with obesity became obese adults, the societal costs over their lifetime might exceed $1.1 Trillion (9).

1. Long-term Trends in Diabetes . (2017, April). Retrieved from https://www.cdc.gov/diabetes/statistics/slides/long_term_trends.pdf

2. Basu, S. et al. (2013, Feb 27). The Relationship of Sugar to Population-Level Diabetes Prevalence: An Econometric Analysis of Repeated Cross-Sectional Data. PLoS ONE 8(2): e57873. Retrieved 2015, from http://journals.plos.org/plosone/article?id=10.1371/journal.pone.0057873

3. American Diabetes Association. (n.d.). Statistics About Diabetes. Retrieved May 27, 2017, from http://www.diabetes.org/diabetes-basics/statistics/

4. National Health Expenditure Projections 2012-2022. (n.d.). Retrieved May 27, 2017, from https://www.cms.gov/Research-Statistics-Data-and-Systems/Statistics-Trends-and-Reports/NationalHealthExpendData/downloads/proj2012.pdf

5. American Heart Association. (n.d.). Overweight & Obesity. Retrieved May 27, 2017, from http://www.heart.org/idc/groups/heart-public/@wcm/@sop/@smd/documents/downloadable/ucm_319588.pdf

6. Thorpe KE, Florence CS, Howard DH, Joski P. Trends: The impact of obesity on rising medical spending. Health Aff 2004;Suppl Web Exclusives:W4-480 –W4-486

7. Moses, H. et al. (2013). The anatomy of health care in the United States. JAMA,310(18), 1947-1963. doi:10.1001/jama.2013.281425

8. Soechtig, S. (Director). (2014, May 9). Fed Up [Video for purchase]. Retrieved from http://fedupmovie.com/#/page/home

9. Matthew Kasman, Ross A. Hammond, Aurite Werman, Austen Mack-Crane, and Robin A. McKinnon. (2015, May 12). An In-Depth Look at the Lifetime Economic Cost of Obesity. Retrieved May 27, 2017, from https://www.brookings.edu/wp-content/uploads/2015/05/0512-Obesity-Presentation-v6-RM.pdf

Cost categories associated with obesity include the following (1):

- Direct medical costs: Costs of health care or medicine owing to obesity

- Productivity cost: Absenteeism-Cost of time away from work owing to obesity

- Productivity cost: Presenteeism-The impact of obesity on reduced productivity at work

- SSDI (Social Security Disability Insurance): Cost of SSDI claimed because of complications arising from obesity

- Short-Term Disability: Cost of short-term disability incurred by private firms because of complications arising from obesity

- Taxes Foregone: Taxes foregone due to lower wages resulting from obesity

Obesity is linked to medical cost increases for individuals, taxpayers, and employers. According to an Emory University study, two trends are represented in this increase: the increase in obesity prevalence and the increase in spending on the obese relative to those in the normal-weight category (2). Three obesity-related conditions, in particular, contribute to obesity-related spending increases. According to the Emory University study, "The rise in obesity contributed to large spending increases for the three medical conditions examined (diabetes, hyperlipidemia, and heart disease) from 1987 to 2001" (2).

The cost projections for diet-driven disease are not set in stone because they are 84% preventable (3). Cost control is

> 84% of healthcare costs are preventable

very much within our reach. Through effective preventative health care, trends in chronic disease related spending can be brought under control.

1. Matthew Kasman, Ross A. Hammond, Aurite Werman, Austen Mack-Crane, and Robin A. McKinnon. (2015, May 12). An In-Depth Look at the Lifetime Economic Cost of Obesity. Retrieved May 27, 2017, from https://www.brookings.edu/wp-content/uploads/2015/05/0512-Obesity-Presentation-v6-RM.pdf

2. Thorpe, K. et al. (2004). The Impact Of Obesity On Rising Medical Spending. Health Aff (Millwood). doi:10.1377/hlthaff.w4.480

3. Moses, H. et al. (2013). The anatomy of health care in the United States. JAMA,310(18), 1947-1963. doi:10.1001/jama.2013.281425

2

HOW DIETARY GUIDELINES HELPED ESTABLISH THE STANDARD AMERICAN DIET AND HOW THEY CAN HELP US CHANGE IT

Why do the U.S. dietary guidelines have a high impact on the general public?

THE U.S. GOVERNMENT has issued dietary guidelines since 1980. They are required by law to be published jointly every 5 years by the Department of Health and Human Services and the USDA (1). The current edition is for 2015–2020. These guidelines are used to develop federal food, nutrition, and health policies and programs. Current revisions in the dietary guidelines are designed to help reverse trends in diet-driven disease. The guidelines have had a massive impact on the general public and the food industry. Businesses, schools, community groups, media, the food industry, and state and local governments all utilize the dietary guidelines to develop programs, policies, and communication (1). The food industry responded to the guidelines and other directives by producing low-fat, high-carbohydrate processed foods. They are still the most prominent items in grocery store aisles.

> Before the arrival of the Western diet, indigenous populations had very low levels of heart disease, diabetes, and cancer

Studies of indigenous populations throughout the world have clarified the role of the western low-fat, high-carb diet. The plus-minus [experiment] of adding and subtracting the Western diet has been performed unintentionally in many indigenous populations. Before the arrival of the Western diet, indigenous populations had very low levels of heart disease, diabetes, and cancer. After a few decades of consuming a low-fat, high-carb Western-style diet, these populations acquired all of these chronic diseases at high levels (2). When people switch off of the western diet, diabetes can be reversed if addressed in the early to middle stages, sometimes even in late stages. Other chronic diseases can improve or reverse to lesser degrees. By subtracting the Western diet and adding a functional medicine diet, thousands of people in America are currently reversing their diabetes and improving comorbidities.

The low-fat, high-carb dogma began picking up momentum in the 1970s (3). Eventually, the original USDA low-fat, high-carb food pyramid arrived. Its daily dietary guidelines were as follows:

- 6–11 servings of bread, rice, pasta, and cereal
- 2–4 servings of fruits, including high-glycemic fruits like bananas and grapes

- 3–5 servings of vegetables, including starchy vegetables like potatoes
- 2–3 servings of meat, fish, poultry, nuts, and eggs
- 2–3 servings of milk, yogurt, and cheese
- Fats and sweets "sparingly"

The USDA food pyramid, the food industry, and leaders in the medical field had enormous influence in establishing a large variety of high-carb, low-fat products. Most people, including medical professionals, believed that high-carb, low-fat was healthy. As a result, almost anything that was low-fat was considered healthy. For example, high-sugar snacks such as SnackWells successfully advertised themselves as low-fat, healthy choices. A wide variety of products considered healthy are not (4):

- Commercial salad dressings
- Fruit juices
- Heart healthy whole wheat
- Margarine
- Sports drinks
- Sweeteners
- Agave nectar
- Brown rice syrup
- Processed foods
  - Protein bars
  - Processed vegan foods
  - Processed organic foods
  - Processed vegetable oils
  - Processed gluten-free foods
  - Processed breakfast cereals

What makes most of these foods unhealthy is their high level of flour, sweeteners, and sugar. High-sugar foods and simple carbohydrates can be portrayed as healthy simply because they are low-fat. This was especially true in the 1980s and 1990s when I used to drink large quantities of fruit juice sweetened with high-fructose corn syrup thinking it was healthy. I reasoned that it was healthy because it was full of vitamin C and low-fat.

1. USA, USDA. (2015). Dietary Guidelines 2015-2020. Retrieved from https://health.gov/dietaryguidelines/2015/guidelines/executive-summary

2. Taubes, G. (2016). *The case against sugar.* New York: Alfred A. Knopf.

3. Teicholz, N. (2014). Big Fat Surprise. New York, NY: Simon and Schuster

4. Spritzler, F. (2016, June 27). 10 "Low-Fat" Foods That Are Actually Bad For You. Retrieved from https://authoritynutrition.com/10-unhealthy-low-fat-foods/

How do the current U.S. dietary guidelines differ from functional medicine recommendations?

The current U.S. dietary guidelines have improved dramatically over previous versions such as the original food pyramid and the modified My Pyramid. There are both significant similarities and differences between U.S. dietary guidelines and other recommendations. A summary is included below (1):

- All healthy diets include vegetables and whole fruits as the main part of meals
  - U.S. dietary guidelines include starchy vegetables
  - Functional medicine guidelines strongly discourage starchy vegetables

- Healthy diets may include grains
  - U.S. dietary guidelines include whole grains and processed grains
  - Functional medicine guidelines include limited whole grains but strongly discourage all processed foods and gluten-containing grains.
- Healthy diets include protein sources such as fish, poultry, lean meat, eggs, nuts, seeds, and legumes
  - U.S. dietary guidelines include soy products
  - Functional medicine guidelines discourage omega-6 containing soy products
- Healthy diets may include dairy products
  - U.S. dietary guidelines include low-fat dairy products
  - Functional medicine guidelines discourage dairy products. Some highly regarded doctors include high-fat dairy products (2)
- All healthy diets limit trans fats
- Healthy diets may include saturated fat
  - U.S. dietary guidelines recommend less than 10% saturated fat in the diet
  - Functional medicine guidelines recommend 25–75% fat-containing diets, including avocado, olive oil, nuts, seeds and saturated fats like coconut oil
- All healthy diets limit sugar intake to low levels (less than 10% of calories).

All healthy diets limit sugar intake to low levels (less than 10% of calories).

1. USA, USDA. (2015). Dietary Guidelines 2015-2020. Retrieved from https://health.gov/dietaryguidelines/2015/guidelines/executive-summary

2. Ludwig, D. (2016). Always Hungry. New York, NY: Grand Central Life and Style.

What strategy do the new U.S. dietary guidelines use to help people improve nutrition?

Overall eating patterns are a strong determinant of health. The dietary guidelines utilize patterns to help people gain momentum in establishing healthy eating behaviors. Accordingly, the dietary guidelines contain suggestions for eating patterns as follows (1):

- Lifespan pattern: Establish a healthy eating pattern across a lifespan.

- Nutrient density pattern: Select a variety of foods that are nutrient dense.

- Low sugar pattern: Eat foods low in sugar and salt.

- Low saturated fat pattern: Eat foods low in saturated fat. This is not recommended by doctors in functional and integrative medicine. They recommend a higher fat intake, including highly saturated fats like coconut oil. At the same time, they discourage consumption of non-organic meat and cured meat high in fat.

- Preference pattern: Include cultural and personal preferences when determining food selections to help you establish a healthy eating pattern.

Daily (unless otherwise noted) dietary guidelines for functional medicine are as follows (2):

- Unlimited amounts of non-starchy vegetables
- 3 to 5 servings of healthy fat
- 4 to 6 ounces of protein per meal
- 1 cup low-glycemic fruits
- Up to 2 servings of starchy vegetables
- Half cup of gluten-free grains
- 1 cup of beans
- Unlimited amounts of spices and herbs
- Recreational treats such as sweets & alcohol sparingly

Gluten and dairy products are absent in the functional medicine diet by Dr. Mark Hyman. In addition, there are major reversals in the amount of fat and starchy carbs recommended between the functional medicine guidelines and the original USDA food pyramid. The Hyman Pegan diet combines elements of paleo diets and vegan diets. The result is a healthy fat diet low in grains and high in non-starchy vegetables. Protein and healthy fat also make significant contributions. Low levels of gluten and dairy decrease inflammatory reactions in the body.

1. USA, USDA. (2015). Dietary Guidelines 2015-2020. Retrieved from https://health.gov/dietaryguidelines/2015/guidelines/executive-summary

2. Mark Hyman, MD. (n.d.). How Our Government Made Us Fat and Sick! Retrieved May 27, 2017, from http://drhyman.com/blog/2016/02/26/how-our-government-made-us-fat-and-sick/

What is the American diet or the Western-style diet that is at the center of global chronic disease?

Major characteristics include:

High levels of:
Simple carbohydrates:

- Soft drinks, desserts, high-sugar snacks and processed foods, bread, rice, pasta, potato, and cereal
- 300 pounds of simple, refined carbs per year per American
- Overconsumption of starchy and simple carbohydrates in the total diet

Processed oils

- Trans fats (hydrogenated)
- Inflammatory omega-6 oils (corn and soybean oil)

Animal protein and fat

- Cured or processed meats (sausage, bacon, deli meats)

Low levels of:

- non-starchy veggies
- fiber
- healthy fat (avocados, nuts, seeds, olive oil)

As mentioned, the historically high consumption of simple carbohydrates has been a major factor in the current epidemics of type 2 diabetes, obesity, and associated diet-driven diseases.

Overconsumption of simple carbs drives cravings, weight gain, and insulin resistance—all major health issues. Research has clarified specific sweeteners that have a higher impact than other consumables. High fructose corn syrup is one of these.

Why is HFCS so bad? The fructose molecules in HFCS are free and unbound as a result of the manufacturing process. In this form, they are ready for absorption and utilization. "In contrast, every fructose molecule in sucrose that comes from cane sugar or beet sugar is bound to a corresponding glucose molecule and must go through an extra metabolic step before it can be utilized" (1).

Rats in a Princeton study became obese by drinking high-fructose corn syrup, but not by drinking sucrose. This may be related to how excess fructose is metabolized to produce fat. Glucose, however, is mostly processed for energy or stored as glycogen in the liver and muscles. According to Dr. Mark Hyman, "Fructose goes right to the liver and triggers lipogenesis (the production of fats like triglycerides and cholesterol). This is why it is the major cause of liver damage in this country and causes a condition called "fatty liver" which affects 70 million people" (2). Since the introduction of high-fructose corn syrup as a cost-effective sweetener over 40 years ago, rates of obesity in the U.S. have risen from 15 percent in 1970 to one-third of the American adults today. Americans consume 60 pounds of HFCS every year.

Carbohydrate intake is one of the main activities responsible for increases in cholesterol in the bloodstream. Fat is not usually responsible for increased cholesterol levels in the bloodstream. This is partly because fat stimulates the least amount of insulin production. Sometimes coconut oil can lead to an increase in cholesterol in the blood. However, it is an increase in light, fluffy LDL particles, not in the dangerous small dense LDL particles (3). The type of cholesterol is much more important than the total cholesterol.

1. Parker, H. (2010, March 22). A sweet problem: Princeton researchers find that high-fructose corn syrup prompts considerably more weight gain. Retrieved June 08, 2017, from https://www.princeton.edu/news/2010/03/22/sweet-problem-princeton-researchers-find-high-fructose-corn-syrup-prompts

2. Hyman, M. (2015, November 11). 5 Reasons High Fructose Corn Syrup Will Kill You. Retrieved June 08, 2017, from http://drhyman.com/blog/2011/05/13/5-reasons-high-fructose-corn-syrup-will-kill-you/

3. Hyman, M. (2017, March 22). Is Coconut Oil Bad for Your Cholesterol? Retrieved June 08, 2017, from http://drhyman.com/blog/2016/04/06/is-coconut-oil-bad-for-your-cholesterol/

Americans consume too much unhealthy fat

Unhealthy fats are also a problem. "A typical North American diet may contain 11 to 30 times more omega-6 fatty acids than omega-3 fatty acids, contributing to the rising rate of inflammatory disorders in the United States" (1). Omega-6 fatty acid is a polyunsaturated fat, essential for human health because it cannot be made in the body. People must obtain omega-6 fatty acids by consuming foods such as meat, poultry, and eggs as well as nut and plant-based oils such as canola and sunflower oils. Healthy diets consist of roughly two to four times more omega-6 fatty acids than omega-3 fatty acids (1). Thus, the American diet has as much as 15 times the recommended level of omega 6 oil. Sources of omega-6 fatty acids include: Soybean oil, Corn oil, Safflower Oil, Sunflower Oil, Peanut Oil, Cottonseed Oil, Rice Bran Oil, Meat, Eggs, and Dairy Products.

Insulin resistance and inflammation are the cellular mechanisms largely responsible for the major global chronic diseases. Insulin-related issues eventually lead to blood vessel leakage and breakdown. Inflammation leads to blood vessel blockage. This combination is powerful but reversible.

The Western-style diet described above interacts with other lifestyle factors. The main components of an unhealthy physical state include:

- Diets high in processed foods and refined carbohydrate.
- Diets with insufficient levels of green leafy vegetables and non-starchy vegetables.
- Diets with low levels of healthy fats
- High levels of unregulated stress
- Insufficient levels of aerobic exercise

What leads to these unhealthy components? Some of the main factors include time limitations, financial limitations, and identity issues. All 3 reinforce each other and increase the overall health impacts. The good news is that three is a reasonable number of issues to address in getting health back on track.

1. Omega-3, 6, and 9 and How They Add Up. (n.d.). Retrieved May 27, 2017, from http://www.uccs. edu/Documents/healthcircle/pnc/health-topics/ Omega-3_6_and_9_Fats.pdf

Turning point in nutrition recommendations and diets

High-carb/low-fat was a pyramid scheme

It is perhaps more accurate to describe the low-fat, high-carb craze of the past several decades as a pyramid scheme than the financial pyramid schemes that took place in the investment business. Most Americans followed food pyramids recommended by the U.S. government.

It was a scheme because these pyramids were based more on politics than science. A few influential scientists pushed the low-fat diet on the government, and the government adopted it (1). The fat research upon which the low-fat, high-carb food pyramid was based was clearly faulty. It was discovered to be faulty because of the results of decades of eating high-carb, low-fat products.

A turning point arrived in 2016 when leading doctors and scientists began making their nutrition findings available to the masses (*Always Hungry*, Ludwig, D.; *Eat Fat, Get Thin*, Hyman, M.). 2015 marked a change in nutritional recommendations from the government that shockingly included the identification of dietary cholesterol as a substance no longer of concern (2,3).

> 2015 marked a change in nutritional recommendations from the government that shockingly included the identification of dietary cholesterol as a substance no longer of concern.

Many people are now aware that high-carb, low-fat diets are not healthy. However, at least two major factors decrease the likelihood of fast dietary changes amongst the population. A food environment saturated with processed foods containing high levels of sugar, flour, and artificial ingredients will not change overnight. In addition, people addicted to eating high-sugar, processed foods will not change their habits overnight. Most people will continue eating these foods even if they know that they are unhealthy. Reducing the consumption of these foods to lower levels will probably be good enough for most. Even those suffering a heart attack do not significantly change their eating habits (4).

For these reasons and others, organizations such as Blue Zones are working to change the food environment and cultural environment. If the food and cultural environment change towards a healthy diet, the chances of more people in the population altering their eating habits improve.

1. Hyman, M. (2016). Eat fat, get thin: why the fat we eat is the key to sustained weight loss and vibrant health. New York: Little, Brown and Company.

2. USA, USDA. (2015). Dietary Guidelines 2015-2020. Retrieved from https://health.gov/dietaryguidelines/2015/guidelines/executive-summary

3. Joseph Mercola . (n.d.). 2015 Dietary Guidelines for Americans Makes Strides Toward Better Nutrition, But Fallacies Remain. Retrieved May 27, 2017, from http://articles.mercola.com/sites/articles/archive/2015/06/1 5/2015-dietary-guidelines.aspx

4. Alyssa Davis. (2015, November 18). Despite Having Heart Attack, Many Smoke, Are Obese. Retrieved May 27, 2017, from http://www.gallup.com/poll/186560/heart-attack-smoke-obese.aspx

Was 2015 the beginning of a major turning point in the American diet?

In recent decades, many doctors believed low-fat nutrition recommendations until they saw so many patients suffering the health consequences of low-fat/ high-carb diets that they began to consider alternatives. It took an epidemic of chronic disease impacting the entire nation to generate the momentum necessary for a wider turning point both in research and eating habits. Yet it's just the beginning of a turning point.

Momentum has been building for several years. Healthy diets in various forms such as the Zone Diet (1), Paleo diet (2), and Mediterranean diet all helped bring greater awareness. All of these diets placed a significant emphasis on non-starchy vegetables and protein and a lowered emphasis on grains. Researchers are now gathering data that will provide the basis of personalized diets, the ultimate diet to optimize health.

1. Barry, S. (n.d.). The Zone Diet. Retrieved June 08, 2017, from http://www.zonediet.com/the-zone-diet/

2. Vandyken, P. (2016, October 12). WHAT TO EAT ON THE PALEO DIET. Retrieved May 27, 2017, from http://thepaleodiet.com/what-to-eat-on-the-pale o-diet-paul-vandyken/

The history of low-fat, high-carb and the government's dietary guidelines

A series of books has documented the historic connection between dietary guidelines and low-fat, high-carb diets. Some of the best are included below. In addition, a history of the USDA dietary guidelines is provided by the government at this link: https://health.gov/dietaryguidelines/history.htm

- Taubes, G. Why We Get Fat is a groundbreaking book making the case that sugar is the tobacco of the new millennium (1):

- Taubes, G. The Case Against Sugar thoroughly investigates Americans' history with sugar and how sugar overconsumption is at the center of chronic disease (2).

- Teicholz, N. The Big Fat Surprise explains the politics, personalities, and history of how Americans came to believe that dietary fat is bad for health (3). The Big Fat Surprise was the first mainstream publication to make the argument for why saturated fats found in dairy, meat, and eggs are not bad for health. The Economist named it the #1 science book of 2014, and it was also named a 2014 *Best Book* by the Wall Street Journal, Forbes, and Mother Jones.

1. Taubes, G. (2011). Why we get fat: and what to do about it. New York: Anchor Books.

2. Taubes, G. (2016). The case against sugar. New York: Alfred A. Knopf.

3. Teicholz, N. (2014). Big Fat Surprise. New York, NY: Simon and Schuster

Are diets in the U.S. changing?

It is sometimes difficult to imagine that the U.S. diet is changing when we are surrounded by fast food and convenience food. Yet it is changing in major ways. Soft drink consumption has been decreasing for 11 consecutive years and 25 years overall. Recently, diet soda sales have experienced dramatic annual drops of up to 6% (2015) (1). The public is increasingly concerned about the health risks associated with artificial sweeteners and the diabetes risk associated with sweetened soft drinks. In response, soft drink companies have been beefing up their non-sweetened beverages. Bottled water consumption has risen 6–11%. It is encouraging that soft drink manufacturers are adapting to the changes and can potentially be drivers for consumption of healthy unsweetened drinks.

Daily consumption of sweetened drinks is a known health hazard, but specific risk quantitation for consumer products is not yet available. It is likely that research will demonstrate specific risk percentages associated with different levels of soft drink consumption. The case against high levels of soft drink consumption may become as strong or stronger than the case against smoking. As a result, the public may one day see organizational policies and public ordinances against soft drink consumption in places such as schools and health conscious organizations. This kind of shift may seem implausible in the wake of the popularization of super-sized drinks. Smoking ordinances also seemed implausible at one time.

Beef production has been decreasing for at least 13 years. The number of cattle harvested has decreased 19% since 2002 (2). This is a large change for a staple component of the standard American diet. America consumes more pounds of meat per capita than any people in the history of the world. Consumption of red meat is in a sustained decline. In 1972, "the average American consumed at least 104 pounds of red meat a year, according to the United States Department of Agriculture." By 2012, that average had fallen to 75 pounds, a drop of more than 25%." All meat consumption, including poultry and fish, has fallen about 10% per capita since 2004 (3).

Health concerns may be the main reason meat consumption is decreasing. A World Health Organization (WHO) report identified processed meat as "carcinogenic." The International Agency for Research on Cancer (IARC), a WHO agency, indicated that there was enough evidence to rank processed meat as a "group 1" cancer-causing agent, a category that includes plutonium, arsenic, and tobacco (3). As little as two slices of bacon per day could increase the risk of colorectal cancer by 18%. In addition, health risks were identified in association with all red meat, concluding that "even the freshest beef, pork and veal is 'probably' a cause of cancer." Findings such as this have significant influence in creating long-term change toward healthier diets.

1. Kell, J. (2016, March 29). Soda Consumption Falls to 30-Year Low In The U.S. Retrieved May 27, 2017, from http://fortune.com/2016/03/29/soda-sales-drop-11th-year/

2. Statistics & Information. (n.d.). Retrieved May 27, 2017, from https://www.ers.usda.gov/topics/animal-products/cattle-beef/statistics-information.aspx

3. World Health Organization, International Agency for Research on Cancer. (2105, October 26). *IARC Monographs evaluate consumption of red meat and processed meat*[Press release]. Retrieved November 1, 2017, from https://www.iarc.fr/en/media-centre/pr/2015/pdfs/pr240_E.pdf

What can the standard American diet change to?

Is traditional American fast-food here to stay: burgers, fries, shakes? It may seem unrealistic for most Americans to give up fast food, processed snacks, and convenience food. However, popular alternatives already exist. Mediterranean-style diets have wide appeal and could transition people to even healthier diets. Alternatively, the Mediterranean diet itself could undergo changes which make it even healthier.

Here are some tips on eating a Mediterranean diet (1):

- Eat seven to ten servings a day of fruits and vegetables
- Eat almonds, cashews, pistachios, and walnuts on hand for a quick snack. Try tahini (blended sesame seeds) as a dip or spread for bread

- Switch from regular pasta and rice to whole-grain varieties

- Replace butter with healthy fats such as olive oil and canola oil

- Use herbs and spices instead of salt to flavor foods. Herbs and spices improve flavor and are rich in health-promoting substances

- Limit red meat to no more than a few times a month. Substitute fish and poultry for red meat. Avoid sausage, bacon, and other high-fat meats

- Eat fish and poultry at least twice a week. Fresh or water-packed tuna, salmon, trout, mackerel, and herring are healthy choices

- Enjoy meals with family and friends

- Get plenty of exercise

1. Mayo Foundation. (n.d.). Mediterranean diet: A heart-healthy eating plan. Retrieved May 27, 2017, from http://www.mayoclinic.org/healthy-lifestyle/nutrition-and-healthy-eating/in-depth/mediterranean-diet/art-20047801?inf_contact_key=87ec195ccf2d1e9fe90e666d21a57f05278923d70eb-fe32d0607eedc35b7900f

The Daniel Plan diet is a delicious way to transition out of the SAD diet

A 68-year-old insulin-dependent type 2 diabetic lost 50 pounds and was able to get off diabetes and blood pressure medication on the 4th day.

The Daniel Plan is another healthy diet that can help people transition out of the standard American diet. Dr. Mark Hyman leads this part of the plan, and he shares his expertise gained over decades of first-hand experience with patients. He has helped thousands reverse chronic diseases such as diabetes, heart disease, and chronic stress. Thousands of people are already following the Eat Fat, Get Thin protocol (1). A 68-year-old insulin-dependent type 2 diabetic lost 50 pounds and was able to get off diabetes and blood pressure medication on the 4th day. He helps thousands of others through his 10 other best-selling health books.

The Daniel Plan diet is rigorous and yet there is significant flexibility to transition from the typical American diet into The Daniel Plan. They call it the 90/10 rule. People can eat recommended food 90% of the time and then splurge on a little dessert or some other off plan item 10% of the time.

The Daniel Plan guidelines include 50% non-starchy vegetables, 25% lean protein, and 25% whole grains and starchy vegetables. In addition, low glycemic fruit and water or herbal tea is recommended. There's a strong emphasis on reducing intake of processed foods, artificial sweeteners, and simple sugars. Included in the Daniel Plan diet is a section on how to reduce cravings. According to Dr. Hyman, "studies show that when you eat healthy fats, you stay full and energized longer, cut cravings and shed excess weight without feeling deprived." This section facilitates transition out of the craving-inducing standard American diet to a healthy fat diet that helps control cravings. It doesn't hurt that the recipes are delicious.

Dr. Hyman even eats dessert.

Some of his personal favorites include:

- Chocolate Raspberry Smoothie
- Savory Coconut Pancakes

- Chicken and Arugula Salad with Roasted Red Pepper Vinaigrette
- Sweet Potato Soup with Coconut and Ginger
- Grilled Red Wine and Rosemary Sirloin Steak with Mushrooms
- No-Bake Walnut Brownies

There are plenty of alternatives to comfort foods, including desserts, that you can indulge in—guilt-free. Another food myth is that it is too expensive to eat healthy. The URL below provides access to the environmental working group's recommendations for eating healthy on a budget (2).

1. Hyman, M.. (n.d.). Eat Fat, Get Thin Course. Retrieved May 27, 2017, from http://drhyman.com/efgt-course/
2. Environmental Working Group. (2012, August). GOOD FOOD ON A TIGHT BUDGET. Retrieved May 27, 2017, from http://www.ewg.org/goodfood/

3

THE PREVENTIVE HEALTH CARE MOVEMENT IS UNDERWAY

AS THE CHANGES in American dietary patterns attest, the preventive health care movement is underway. Practical and personal reasons demand it. As mentioned, the current burden of chronic disease is not sustainable either individually or collectively. Preventive health care should start with what we already know will help people become healthier such as healthy diet and lifestyle. Although screening for specific diseases is an excellent way to prevent their advancement, a number of people tested, about one in three men, have no regular doctor (1). No one knows how many people put off medical visits or whether it is harmful. National statistics do not currently track delays in care.

1. Sandman, D. et al. (2000, March). OUT OF TOUCH: AMERICAN MEN AND THE HEALTH CARE SYSTEM. Retrieved May 27, 2017, from http://www.commonwealthfund.org/~/media/files/publications/fund-report/2000/mar/

out-of-touch--american-men-and-the-health-care-system/
sandman_outoftouch_374-pdf.pdf

What works for physical health?

The main issues involved in an unhealthy lifestyle include unregulated stress, eating the wrong foods, and lack of exercise. The reverse of these can restore physical health if supported by a community of relationships and good non-physical health.

A healthy diet can be summarized simply:

- dominant in non-starchy vegetables
- healthy fats such as olive oil, coconut oil, nuts, and seeds
- modest amounts of lean protein
- elimination of 90% or more of refined carbohydrates and processed foods

What is the technological foundation for personalized medicine?

There have been a number of periods throughout history where scientific advancement has exploded. However, we probably live in the most exciting time of scientific discovery yet. Astounding findings in basic research are emerging from biology, physics, and cosmology. In applied science, nutrition and preventive health care are some of the most exciting fields. It is particularly exciting that genetically fine-tuned, maximized health will be within our reach in the coming decades.

Dr. Craig Venter led one of the two scientific groups that originally sequenced the human genome. His group, Celera Genomics, sequenced the human genome for $100 million dollars with a building-sized $50 million computer. The federal government also sequenced the human genome at the same time with a different strategy which cost $2.7 billion dollars (1). Although both projects returned great value on the investment, the ability of technology to increase efficiency and cut costs is obvious. The current standard for human genome cost is $2,000 per genome (2). This is over 1 million fold less than the original cost. Technological advances achieved this million-fold cost decrease in 13 years. It is projected that sequencing costs will drop to $100 per genome in the near future, resulting in a 20-million-fold cost decrease.

This low DNA sequencing cost is highly advantageous for gathering the data needed for personalized medicine. Venter's latest goal is to sequence the genomes of 1 million people over the next 10 years and combine it with the donor's health histories and medical test results in order to diagnose, treat, and prevent a range of disorders, including chronic diseases such as cancer, diabetes, and heart disease. The availability of such large volumes of genetic data enables the determination of rare genetic variants involved in disease pathogenesis. This, in turn, will elucidate the genetic markers needed for personalized medicine. For example, if a patient has markers for hypercholesterolemia, their diet can be adjusted accordingly. Since nutritional science is gaining momentum, it is anticipated that many significant studies will emerge that use genomic information and other test results to elucidate the impact of a wide variety of dietary components on human health. It should be possible to test an individual for the characteristics that determine their optimal diet. Since the central components of the top chronic diseases are diet-driven, optimized diets have the capacity to relieve significant proportions of the global healthcare burden.

> The cost of DNA sequencing has dropped 20 million fold.

1. National Human Genome Research Institute. (2010, October 30). Human Genome Project Completion: Frequently Asked Questions. Retrieved May 27, 2017, from https://www.genome.gov/11006943/human-genome-project-completion-frequently-asked-questions/

2. Weintraub, A. (2016). Craig Venter's latest production. Technology Review,119(5), 94-95.

What are the advantages of optimized diets?

> People engaging in healthy lifestyles save themselves and the community up to 50% of their lifetime health care costs.

The best way to focus personalized medicine is on preventive health care. People engaging in healthy lifestyles save themselves and the community up to 50% of their lifetime health care costs. (1) Few other initiatives can free up this magnitude of financial and human resources. Healthy people save the community money and increase productivity generating more sustainable communities.

DNA sequencing data from millions of different people potentially allows a new generation of genetic testing that can optimize diet and deliver results of unparalleled accuracy. Advantages of optimized diets may include:

- Prevention of chronic diseases: Diabetes, heart disease, cancer, Alzheimer's, and others

- Treatment of chronic diseases: Diabetes, heart disease, cancer, Alzheimer's, and others,

- Maximized personal energy

- Maximized mental clarity
- Negation of the need for medication

Results such as those listed above are currently happening as a result of conversion to healthy lifestyles. Personalized diets should magnify this effect.

1. The impact of wellness on community sustainability [Interview by T. Schierer]. (2016, November). JETT Radio interview with Dr. Mike Roizen https://vimeo.com/193400128

Exercise is the one thing that helps everything

Exercises needs a flexible approach. Most important is for people to find an exercise program that works for them even if it is very unconventional. Finding ways to move throughout the day such as taking the stairs can make the difference in building a healthy exercise program that works. Regulating stress is mainly a function of regulating the thoughts and beliefs that generate stress. This thought regulation makes way for new beliefs that lower stress.

The exercise portion of The Daniel Plan (DP) describes the advantages of exercise, including energy enhancement, improve sleep quality, and a host of other benefits. As with the DP diet, flexibility makes The Daniel Plan exercise components more likely to succeed. They provide guidelines instead of a rigid system. The plan includes finding a form of exercise that works with the individual's motivation so that they can do it consistently. Suggestions include exercising with a group, including a variety of different exercises and starting at a level that does not lead to burnout. It also helps to find ways to move throughout the day that are part of a person's normal routine, finding movement that is enjoyable and motivational to the individual, and including warm-ups and stretching breaks.

Advantages of exercise noted by The Daniel Plan include:

- increasing lung capacity muscle tone and blood flow
- brain stimulation sharpening listening skills improving problem-solving skills
- delaying age-associated memory loss
- creation of relationships
- reduction of risk for diabetes and high cholesterol
- lowering risk of heart disease and cancer and osteoporosis
- strengthening of the immune system
- decrease levels of depression stress and anxiety
- increase fat burning
- improved sleep
- improved energy
- improved productivity

Given this long list of benefits, it's no wonder that Dr. Mark Hyman describes exercise as the one thing that helps everything.

1. Warren, R. et al. (2013). *The Daniel plan: 40 days to a healthier life*. Grand Rapids, MI: Zondervan.

Cancer as a model for prevention

Cancer and heart disease are diet-driven chronic diseases related to diabetes and obesity. While type 2 diabetes and obesity are the easiest to reverse and can serve as models of the reversal process, cancer and heart disease illustrate prevention well.

Personalized medicine may bring cancer and heart disease farther into the reversal realm. Currently, cancer and heart disease are examples that reversal can sometimes occur in advanced disease states even for diseases that cause a high degree of damage.

Cancer is one of the most misunderstood chronic diseases. It is thought of by many to be a genetic disease, and it is. Cancer is typically a disease of older individuals because it takes decades for enough mutations to accumulate to generate cancerous cells. However, the generation of cancerous cells is highly dependent on behavior. The majority of cancer is preventable. Smoking, pollution, obesity, viral infections from sexually transmitted diseases, and unhealthy diet are among the preventable causes of cancer.

According to the NIH, 90–95% of cancer is preventable because these cases are based on the environment and lifestyle (1). A disease that can often be thought of as incurable is actually highly preventable. Other chronic diseases such as heart disease and stroke are at least 80% preventable (2). Type 2 diabetes is 100% preventable. It would not exist if all people ate a healthy diet.

The genetic changes that result in tumor cells are mostly preventable. According to the NIH, "only 5–10% of all cancer cases can be attributed to congenital defects" (1). This is why it is important to discuss activities that can lead to cancer-producing mutations. These lifestyle factors identified by the NIH include (1):

> The majority of chronic disease is 80-100% preventable

- Cigarette smoking
- Diet (fried foods, red meat)

- Alcohol
- Sun exposure
- Environmental pollutants
- Infections
- Stress
- Obesity
- Physical inactivity

In terms of the death rate per risk factor, the evidence indicates that of all cancer-related deaths, almost 25–30% are due to tobacco, as many as 30–35% are linked to diet, about 15–20% are due to infections, and the remaining percentage are due to other factors like radiation, stress, physical activity, and environmental pollutants. Since we know the risk factors for cancer, we can decrease the risk by reversing these risk factors.

1. Anand, P. et al. (2008). Cancer is a Preventable Disease that Requires Major Lifestyle Changes. *Pharm Res.,25*(9), 2097-2116. doi:10.1007/s11095-008-9661-9

2. Overview - Preventing chronic diseases: a vital investment. (n.d.). Retrieved May 27, 2017, from http://www.who.int/chp/chronic_disease_report/part1/en/index11.html

How to prevent cancer

Most of the main risk factors for cancer are known and preventable. This is the kind of problem that can be turned into a solution. If the problem is preventable, it is not necessarily a problem. The issue then becomes choosing the most effective prevention strategy. With cancer risk factors, the solutions are fairly simple but not easy. Cancer prevention requires:

- smoking cessation
- increased ingestion of fruits and vegetables
- moderate use of alcohol
- caloric restriction
- exercise
- avoidance of direct exposure to sunlight
- minimal meat consumption
- use of whole grains
- use of vaccinations
- regular check-ups

The percentage of cancer-related deaths attributable to diet and tobacco is as high as 60–70% worldwide. Most risk factors for cancer, including cigarette smoke, obesity, alcohol, hyperglycemia, infectious agents, sunlight, stress, food carcinogens, and environmental pollutants, have been shown to activate a molecule called NF-κB (1). NF-κB activation has been encountered in most types of cancers, and it is a mediator of inflammation. In most cancers, chronic inflammation precedes tumorigenesis. The researchers authoring this prevention study conclude that all lifestyle factors that cause cancer and all agents that prevent cancer are linked through chronic inflammation. Specific risk factors are explored in more detail below.

1. Anand, P. et al. (2008). Cancer is a Preventable Disease that Requires Major Lifestyle Changes. *Pharm Res.,25*(9), 2097-2116. doi:10.1007/s11095-008-9661-9

How to prevent cancer: Diet

Diet contributes to cancer risk to varying degrees depending on the type of cancer. It is as high as 70% for colorectal cancer and in about 30 to 35% of cancer deaths overall in the USA (1).

Some of the carcinogens found in our food include:

- Nitrates
- Nitrosamines
- Pesticides
- Dioxins
- Food additives

Nitrites and nitrates are used in meat because they inhibit botulinum exotoxin production. Unfortunately, they are also powerful carcinogens. According to researchers, long-term exposure to food additives such as nitrite preservatives and azo dyes has been associated with cancer (2). Plastic food containers are also a risk. Bisphenol from the plastic can migrate into food and may increase the risk of breast (3) and prostate (4,5) cancers. Types of foods associated with cancer include saturated fatty acids, trans fatty acids, refined sugars and flour present in most processed foods. In addition, food carcinogens have been shown to activate inflammatory pathways, an important factor in the development of cancer.

Heavy consumption of red meat is a risk factor for several cancers, especially for those of the gastrointestinal tract. The list also includes (2): colorectal, prostate, bladder, breast, gastric, pancreatic, and oral cancers. "The heterocyclic amines produced during the cooking of meat are carcinogens. Charcoal cooking and/or smoke curing of meat produces harmful carbon compounds such as pyrolysates and amino acids, which have a strong cancerous effect" (2).

1. Doll, R. and Peto, R. (1981). The causes of cancer: quantitative estimates of avoidable risks of cancer in the United States today. J. Natl. Cancer Inst.,66(6), 1191-308.

2. Anand, P. et al. (2008). Cancer is a Preventable Disease that Requires Major Lifestyle Changes. Pharm Res.,25(9), 2097-2116. doi:10.1007/s11095-008-9661-9

3. Sasaki, Y. F. et al. (2002). The comet assay with 8 mouse organs: results with 39 currently used food additives. Mutat. Res.,519, 103-119.

4. Durando, M. et al. (2007). Prenatal bisphenol A exposure induces preneoplastic lesions in the mammary gland in Wistar rats. Environ. Health Perspect.,115, 80-86.

5. Ho, S. et al. (2006). Developmental exposure to estradiol and bisphenol A increases susceptibility to prostate carcinogenesis and epigenetically regulates phosphodiesterase type 4 variant 4. Cancer Res.,66, 5624-5632. doi:10.1158/0008-5472. CAN-06-0516

How to prevent cancer: weight loss

Obesity has been associated with increased mortality from cancers of the (1):

- Colon
- Breast
- Endometrium
- Kidneys
- Esophagus
- Gastric cardia

- Pancreas
- Prostate
- Gallbladder
- Liver

"In the USA overweight and obesity could account for 14% of all deaths from cancer in men and 20% of those in women" (1). Studies have shown that the common denominators between obesity and cancer include:

- insulin-like growth factor 1 (hormone)
- insulin
- insulin resistance
- inflammation
- other factors, including neurochemicals, leptin, sex steroids, adiposity

Note that 3 of the factors are related directly to insulin. Insulin spikes are generated by high-carb intake. Replacing carbs with non-starchy vegetables is a way to lower cancer risk. High blood glucose often associated with type 2 diabetes and obesity has been shown to activate NF-κB (2), a molecule which could link obesity with cancer. Obesity is a serious condition because of the hormonal implications and imbalances generated as a person becomes obese.

1. Anand, P. et al. (2008). Cancer is a Preventable Disease that Requires Major Lifestyle Changes. *Pharm Res.,25*(9), 2097-2116. doi:10.1007/s11095-008-9661-9

2. Nareika, A. Y. et al. (2008). High glucose enhances lipopolysaccharide-stimulated CD14 expression in U937 mononuclear cells by increasing nuclear factor kappaB and AP-1 activities. *J. Endocrinol.,196*, 45-55. doi:10.1677/ JOE-07-0145

How to prevent cancer: cleaner environments and organic food

Many types of environmental pollution have been linked to various cancers, including (1):

- outdoor air pollution by carbon particles associated with polycyclic aromatic hydrocarbons (PAHs)

- indoor air pollution by environmental tobacco smoke, formaldehyde, and volatile organic compounds such as benzene and 1,3-butadiene (which may particularly affect children)

- food pollution by food additives and by carcinogenic contaminants such as nitrates, pesticides, dioxins, and other organochlorines; carcinogenic metals and metalloids; pharmaceutical medicines; and cosmetics (2)

Numerous outdoor air pollutants such as PAHs increase the risk of cancers. PAHs penetrate our bodies primarily through breathing. They are carried into our bodies by adhering to fine carbon particles in the atmosphere. "Long-term exposure to PAH-containing air in polluted cities was found to increase the risk of lung cancer deaths" (1). Another environmental pollutant, nitric oxide, was found to increase the risk of lung cancer in a European study.

Other air pollution studies have shown (1):

- nitric oxide can induce lung cancer and promote metastasis

- motor vehicle exhaust can increase the risk of childhood leukemia

- dioxan, an environmental pollutant from incinerators, was found to increase the risk of sarcoma and lymphoma

- indoor air pollutants such as volatile organic compounds and pesticides increase the risk of:
  - childhood leukemia and lymphoma
  - brain tumors
  - Wilm's tumors
  - Ewing's sarcoma
  - germ cell tumors

Food pollution studies have shown that long-term exposure to chlorinated drinking water has been associated with increased risk of cancer. "Nitrates, in drinking water, can transform to mutagenic N-nitroso compounds, which increase the risk of lymphoma, leukemia, colorectal cancer, and bladder cancer" (2).

1. Anand, P. et al. (2008). Cancer is a Preventable Disease that Requires Major Lifestyle Changes. *Pharm Res.,25*(9), 2097-2116. doi:10.1007/s11095-008-9661-9

2. Belpomme, D. et al. (2007). The multitude and diversity of environmental carcinogens. *Environ. Res.,105*, 414-429. doi:10.1016/j.envres.2007.07.002

How does disease screening fit into preventative healthcare strategies?

> Early stage type 2 diabetes is the most reversible of all major chronic diseases

Because a large number of people do not see their doctor on a regular basis, it lowers the impact level of health testing as a strategy for preventative health care. About one-third of men do not see their doctor on a regular basis (1). However, targeted screening for the central components of major chronic disease, type 2 diabetes and obesity, can increase the impact of disease screening on preventative healthcare.

Disease screening is important for public health. Without screening, the prevalence of important diseases is not known. Prevalence metrics allow public health officials to plan budgets, target high prevalence areas, and determine best practices and strategies.

Type 2 diabetes is perhaps the most important major chronic disease to screen for because (2):

- It has a central role in all the top chronic diseases: heart disease, cancer, and Alzheimer's.

- Besides obesity, it is the most dependent on food. Given the difficulty in managing body weight and that many obese people reverse diabetes while still obese, type 2 diabetes in it's early stages is the most reversible of all the major chronic diseases.

- It creates an environment that drives other major chronic diseases such as heart disease, cancer, and Alzheimer's.

- If you reverse diabetes, you can make progress in combating other chronic diseases.

- Prediabetes or diabetes impacts 50% of the population (3).

Screening for type 2 diabetes is relatively inexpensive, facilitating a potentially broad impact. The meters are widely available at stores such as Walgreens.

1. Epstein, R. (2000, October 31). Major Medical Mystery: Why People Avoid Doctors. Retrieved May 27, 2017,

from http://www.nytimes.com/2000/10/31/health/major-medical-mystery-why-people-avoid-doctors.html

2. Taubes, G. (2016). *The case against sugar*. New York: Alfred A. Knopf.

3. Menke, A. et al. (2015). Prevalence of and Trends in Diabetes Among Adults in the United States, 1988-2012. *JAMA,314*(10), 1021-1029. doi:10.1001/jama.2015.10029

Who benefits the most financially from preventative health care savings?

According to Dr. Mike Roizen of the Cleveland Clinic, reducing the current burden of chronic disease is the toughest challenge America has faced because Americans are programmed for the short term. One of his main concerns is getting healthcare costs under control before they become unaffordable. He estimates that the tax rate would need to be doubled by 2025 to pay for chronic disease care. It will a require a "total effort" by Americans much like World War 2 to become healthy as a nation. It is possible that significant rationing of medicine could take place (1).

End of life healthcare costs do not make up the majority of the highest healthcare expenditures. Researchers found that among those with the highest costs, "only 11% were in their last year of life, and approximately 13% of the $1.6 trillion spent on personal health care costs in the United States was devoted to care of individuals in their last year of life" (2).

End of life medical costs are disproportionately high for those with long-term chronic disease and a functional limitation. Some limitations are associated with preventable chronic disease, and others are unavoidable due to genetic defects. Data suggest that significant health care cost savings could be realized through screening of preventable chronic diseases such as type 2 diabetes, heart disease, cancer, and Alzheimer's.

Positive results can be obtained by implementing preventive measures for those who have not acquired a chronic disease and by implementing rehabilitative measures for those with discrete high-cost events such as a heart attack or cancer diagnosis. Patients compliant with rehabilitative health and lifestyle changes can return to stable health with low healthcare costs.

Untreated chronic disease results in high end of life health-care costs and a substantial portion of overall health care costs. A recent analysis of US health care spending revealed that chronic illnesses account for 84% of total health care costs (3). Reversing this through healthy lifestyle represents our greatest potential source of healthcare cost savings. If preventative healthcare gets reimbursed by insurers, it helps healthcare providers transition from treatment orientation to preventative health care orientation. Long term contracts with patients that provide incentives for a healthy lifestyle will also facilitate this transition.

1. How healthcare impacts community sustainability [Interview by T. Schierer]. (2016, December 28). Interview with Dr. Mike Roizen at the Cleveland Clinic.

2. Aldridge, M. D., & Kelley, A. S. (2015). The Myth Regarding the High Cost of End-of-Life Care. Am J Public Health. ,105(12), 2411-2415. doi:10.2105/ AJPH.2015.302889

3. Moses, H. et al. (2013). The anatomy of health care in the United States. JAMA,310(18), 1947-1963. doi:10.1001/jama.2013.281425

How to screen for chronic disease

As mentioned, diabetes and obesity reside in the center of the main group of chronic diseases that are leading causes of death in the U.S. Testing programs for chronic disease can be simplified by a focus on these central components. Obesity can be determined by weighing individuals and comparing it to a BMI chart. Those with a BMI higher than 30 are considered obese. Diabetes screening is of broader scope than obesity because diabetes testing more closely identifies those who are metabolically obese. Metabolic obesity includes people whose physical weight is normal (MONW) and those who are physically overweight. Obesity only addressed those who are physically overweight.

The concept that some non-obese or slightly obese individuals have several risk factors for metabolic disorders was first proposed by Ruderman et al. ~30 years ago (1). Ongoing investigations reveal that these metabolically obese but normal-weight (MONW) individuals, also called metabolically abnormal normal weight or normal weight obesity, are not uncommon. About 40% of non-obese are metabolically obese (2, 3, 4).

1. Ruderman, N. B. et al. (1981). The 'metabolically-obese,' normal-weight individual. *Am J Clin Nutr.,34*, 1617-1621.

2. Soechtig, S. (Director). (2014, May 9). *Fed Up* [Video file]. Retrieved from http://fedupmovie.com/#/page/home

3. Meigs, J. et al. (2006). Body mass index, metabolic syndrome, and risk of type 2 diabetes or cardiovascular disease. *J Clin Endocrinol Metab.,91*, 2906-2912.

4. Lee, S. et al. (2011). Identifying metabolically obese but normal-weight (MONW) individuals in a nondiabetic Korean population: the Chungju Metabolic disease Cohort (CMC) study. *Clin Endocrinol (Oxf),75*, 475-481.

Metabolic obesity has been defined by at least 3 different criteria (1):

1. Having metabolic syndrome (metabolic syndrome criterion below).

2. Having a TyG index higher than the cutoff value (TyG criterion).

    o Simplified definition of metabolic syndrome: Individuals with a higher TyG index (above 8.82 for men and 8.73 for women) and normal weight (BMI ⩾18.5 and <25 kg m−2) can be classified into the MONW group. This novel criterion successfully reflected the metabolic phenotype of MONW and predicted the future development of diabetes.

    ▪ The TyG index was calculated by the logarithm of fasting triglyceride x fasting glucose divided by 2 (2).

3. Having a homeostasis model assessment (3) estimate of insulin resistance in the highest quartile were designated as MONW.

    ▪ Comparison of a patient's fasting values with the model's predictions allows a quantitative assessment of the contributions of insulin resistance and deficient β-cell function to the fasting hyperglycemia (high blood glucose).

Subjects not fulfilling the above criteria are identified as metabolically healthy and normal weight (MHNW). Measuring the degree of insulin resistance or adiposity are the core characteristics of MONW. A consensus is still lacking, but the existing options are related closely enough so that there is not that much difference (1). Measuring the degree of insulin resistance or belly fat are the core characteristic of MONW. Fat deposits hidden in the white fat that lies around their vital organs, streaked through their underused muscles, and wrapped around the heart can send out the chemical signals which eventually lead to insulin resistance, diabetes, and heart conditions. A few extra pounds of belly weight, while remaining otherwise lean, can signify you are an MONW (4). About 85 percent of people who have type 2 diabetes—the most common type of diabetes—also have metabolic syndrome. These people have a much higher risk for heart disease than the 15 percent of people who have type 2 diabetes without metabolic syndrome (1).

1. Lee, S. et al. (2015). A novel criterion for identifying metabolically obese but normal weight individuals using the product of triglycerides and glucose. *Nutr Diabetes.,5*(4). doi:10.1038/nutd.2014.46

2. Simental-Mendía, L. et al. (2008). The product of fasting glucose and triglycerides as surrogate for identifying insulin resistance in apparently healthy subjects. *Metab Syndr Relat Disord.,6*(4), 299-304. doi:10.1089/met.2008.0034.

3. Matthews, D. et al. (1985). Homeostasis model assessment: insulin resistance and β-cell function from fasting plasma glucose and insulin concentrations in man. *Diabetologia,28*(7), 412-419. doi:10.1007/BF00280883

4. Hyman, M. (n.d.). Why "Skinny Fat" Can Be Worse than Obesity [Web log post]. Retrieved June 8, 2017, from http://drhyman.com/blog/2015/07/16/why-skinny-fat-can-be-worse-than-obesity/

How is metabolic syndrome defined?

Metabolic syndrome is defined as having 3 of the 5 NIH criteria below (1). Since only 1 of the 5 is directly dependent on a weight measurement, this definition allows for metabolically obese, normal weight individuals.

- A Large Waistline - Having a large waistline means that you carry excess weight around your waist (abdominal obesity)
    - A waist measurement of 35 inches or more for women or 40 inches or more for men is a metabolic risk factor. A large waistline means you're at increased risk for heart disease and other health problems.
- A High Triglyceride Level
    - Triglycerides are a type of fat found in the blood. A triglyceride level of 150 mg/dL or higher (or being on medicine to treat high triglycerides) is a metabolic risk factor. (The mg/dL is milligrams per deciliter—the units used to measure triglycerides.)
- A Low HDL Cholesterol Level
    - HDL cholesterol sometimes is called "good" cholesterol. This is because it helps remove cholesterol from your arteries.
    - An HDL cholesterol level of less than 50 mg/dL for women and less than 40 mg/dL for men (or being on medicine to treat low HDL cholesterol) is a metabolic risk factor.
- High Blood Pressure
- A blood pressure of 130/85 mmHg or higher (or being on medicine to treat high blood pressure) is a metabolic risk factor.
    - If only one of your two blood pressure numbers is high, you're still at risk for metabolic syndrome.

- High Fasting Blood Sugar
  - o A normal fasting blood sugar level is less than 100 mg/dL. A fasting blood sugar level between 100–125 mg/dL is considered prediabetes. A fasting blood sugar level of 126 mg/dL or higher is considered diabetes.
  - o A fasting blood sugar level of 100 mg/dL or higher (or being on medicine to treat high blood sugar) is a metabolic risk factor.

"Metabolically obese but normal weight (MONW) individuals constitute a subgroup of normal weight individuals that display impaired insulin sensitivity with a higher risk of developing diabetes, cardiovascular disease and mortality" (2). MONW, who have a normal weight and TyG levels higher than the cutoff, displayed a metabolically unhealthy phenotype and an approximately twofold higher risk of developing diabetes compared with metabolically healthy normal-weight subjects.

1. National Institutes of Health. (n.d.). What is Metabolic Syndrome? Retrieved May 27, 2017, from https://www.nhlbi.nih.gov/health/health-topics/topics/ms/diagnosis

2. Lee, S. et al. (2015). A novel criterion for identifying metabolically obese but normal weight individuals using the product of triglycerides and glucose. *Nutr Diabetes.*,5(4). doi:10.1038/nutd.2014.46

Screening strategy for preventative healthcare

A two-stage screening strategy could effectively and quickly address the most common chronic diseases. It can be summarized as follows:

Stage 1:

- 1 minute: Visual or scale identification of obesity and waist measurement

- 1–2 minutes: Blood pressure

- 2–5 minutes: Fasting blood glucose

- 1–5-minute questionnaire with doctor or health coach, including a determination of the patient's level of willingness to address health concerns

In roughly 10 minutes, people can be screened to identify those likely to have metabolic syndrome. Metabolic syndrome increases their risk of diabetes, heart disease, and stroke (1). In this same short period of time, those ready to take immediate action for their health can be identified. Those not ready to take immediate action can be placed in a nurture program that plants informational seeds of knowledge that increase their awareness over time.

Stage 2 can encompass a more rigorous profile of testing that fine tunes the process of reversing metabolic syndrome.

Stage 2:

- Weight monitoring on a regular schedule

- Blood profile, including triglycerides, HDL, blood sugar tests, and insulin resistance monitoring on a regular schedule

- Health coaching on a weekly or biweekly basis

All of the tests above can be done quickly and are readily available.

Gallup-Healthways can play a significant role in screening physical and nonphysical health through their survey system (2). The Healthways Well-Being Index (WBI) is a measure how respondents are faring in all aspects of their lives: physically, emotionally, socially, and professionally. It also measures how Americans rate the overall quality of their current life and outlook for the future. The WBI began in 2008 and is the largest database of behavioral economics and information concerning holistic well-being in existence. The WBI is calculated on a scale of 0 to 100, where a score of 100 represents ideal well-being.

Gallup interviews random population samples of adults aged 18 and older living in all 50 states and the District of Columbia Gallup. At least 500 U.S. people are interviewed daily. More than 175,000 respondents are interviewed each year, and over 2 million interviews have been conducted to date since 2008.

Findings from the Gallup-Healthways Well-Being Index can be found in weekly, monthly, quarterly, and yearly publications, and by region, state, and community, as appropriate on Gallup. com. To get the full trends for U.S. well-being data collected through the Gallup-Healthways Well-Being Index since 2008, subscribe to Gallup Analytics. Public health data such as this can identify regions needing more assistance with chronic disease. It provides tools to local authorities that facilitate strategic planning to improve the health of their community.

1. National Institutes of Health. (n.d.). What is Metabolic Syndrome? Retrieved May 27, 2017, from https://www. nhlbi.nih.gov/health/health-topics/topics/ms/diagnosis

2. Gallup. (n.d.). How Does the Gallup-Sharecare Well-Being Index Work? . Retrieved June 8, 2017, from http://www. gallup.com/185471/gallup-healthways-index-work. aspx?utm_source=METHODOLOGY&utm_ medium=topic&utm_campaign=tiles

4

CHRONIC DISEASE INTERACTIONS

Hypertension, diabetes, and obesity have global impact on the body and the world population

HYPERTENSION, DIABETES, AND obesity all illustrate how chronic diseases interact in multiple ways. The commonalities of these global impactors include:

- diet-driven
- reinforcing risk factors
- shared risk factors
- asymptomatic in the beginning
- overlapping impacts

Stress could be added to this list except for its noticeable and immediate symptoms. Stress has the added negative of directly impacting mental, emotional, relational, and spiritual health.

How do different types of chronic disease interact?

Most disease problems throughout the world are chronic diseases such as obesity, diabetes, heart disease, and cancer driven by diet and lifestyle. Broad-spectrum chronic diseases are important to identify. Diseases that interact with most of the other chronic diseases are the keys to disease onset and reversal for most of the world. The advantage of a diet driven condition that facilitates several other adverse conditions is that this effect can be reversed. Scientists analyze the broadness of impact of chronic diseases interactions through molecular, genetic, and population studies. Reversibility can be analyzed by the degree of dependency on diet. Doctors all over the country are verifying this relationship between reversibility and diet dependency. They are witnessing dramatic reversals of diabetes and obesity in weeks and months even after decades of unhealthy lifestyle habits. For example, Dean Ornish, MD, has helped heart transplant patients reverse heart disease to the point that they no longer needed a transplant. However, this is probably not due to diet alone (1). Diabetes and obesity will form the central discussion in this section since these conditions are the most reversible and interact with all the major diseases.

1. Teicholz, N. (2014). Big Fat Surprise. New York, NY: Simon and Schuster, Chapter 7

Type 2 diabetes and obesity are at the center of diet-driven disease

Heart disease, Alzheimer's, and cancer are all related to and interact with type 2 diabetes and obesity. Type 2 diabetes and obesity are at the center of chronic diet-driven disease because:

- Both have a central role in all the major chronic diseases: heart disease, cancer, and Alzheimer's.

- Both are highly dependent on food and therefore are the most reversible. Many people reverse diabetes before obesity such as those receiving gastric bypass surgery.

- Both create an environment that drives other major chronic diseases: heart disease, cancer, and Alzheimer's.

- If you reverse diabetes and obesity, you increase your chances of preventing or reversing other chronic diseases.

- Both have high prevalence:
  - Prediabetes or diabetes impacts 50% of the population (1).
  - Obesity impacts 69% of the population (3).

The prevalence of diabetes-related chronic diseases such as heart disease, cancer, and obesity is high. Many adults have more than one chronic disease, and these diseases interact (1). The CDC estimates that one of four adults had two or more chronic health conditions (2).

> Type 2 diabetes and obesity create an environment that drives heart disease, cancer and Alzheimer's.

1. Menke, A. et al. (2015). Prevalence of and Trends in Diabetes Among Adults in the United States, 1988-2012. JAMA,314(10), 1021-1029. doi:10.1001/jama.2015.10029

2. National Institute of Diabetes and Digestive and Kidney Diseases. (n.d.). Overweight & Obesity Statistics. Retrieved May 29, 2017, from https://www.niddk.nih.gov/health-information/health-statistics/overweight-obesity

Does obesity cause type 2 diabetes?

The relationship between obesity and diabetes is not well understood. People who are not overweight can still get type 2 diabetes because it is mostly dependent on the types of food consumed. Thin people with a high intake of simple carbohydrates and high genetic susceptibility to diabetes are known to acquire type 2 diabetes. Obesity is a major risk factor for the development of type 2 diabetes and cardiovascular disease, but it does not cause diabetes (1). Obesity is a risk factor because it is commonly associated with insulin resistance and hyperinsulinemia.

The diabetes risk associated with obesity is probably related most strongly to the types of food consumed by obese individuals. A study by Weyer et al. suggests that obesity is more of a secondary or complicating factor than a direct cause (1). The direct cause of type 2 diabetes remains an overconsumption of simple carbohydrates. Obese individuals tend to overconsume simple carbohydrates. In addition, fat tissue is known to express and secrete a variety of metabolites, hormones, and cytokines that have been implicated in the development of insulin resistance and atherosclerosis. "The molecular basis for the link between obesity, diabetes, and cardiovascular disease remains poorly understood (1)."

1. Weyer, C. et al. (2001). Hypoadiponectinemia in Obesity and Type 2 Diabetes: Close Association with Insulin Resistance and Hyperinsulinemia. J Clin Endocrinol Metab,86(5), 1930-1935. doi:10.1210/jcem.86.5.7463

What connects obesity to heart disease and other chronic conditions?

Obesity corresponds to a sub-clinical inflammatory condition that promotes the production of pro-inflammatory factors involved in the pathogenesis of heart disease and diabetes. Inflammation promotes the formation of plaques on arterial walls and insulin resistance. In advanced patients, a spectrum of chronic diseases related to inflammation develops.

How does inflammation promote the formation of plaques on arterial walls? Obesity chronically activates the innate immune system, resulting in low-grade inflammation of white adipose (fat) tissue (WAT). In obese people, WAT is characterized by an increased production and secretion of a wide range of inflammatory molecules (1).

When the arterial wall becomes inflamed, it expresses adhesion molecules that bind white blood cells. White blood cells then bind to the arterial walls, beginning a process of plaque accumulation and rupture that can eventually block the arterial wall (2). Weight loss can reduce inflammation, and it targets the behaviors that lead to inflammation.

1. Bastard, J. P. et al. (2006). Recent advances in the relationship between obesity, inflammation, and insulin resistance. *Eur Cytokine Netw., 17*(1), 4-12. Retrieved from https://www.ncbi.nlm.nih.gov/pubmed/16613757.

2. Libby, P. et al. (2002). Inflammation and Atherosclerosis. *Circulation, 105*, 1135-1143. doi:10.1161/hc0902.104353

What is the link between diabetes, heart disease, and stroke?

High blood glucose from diabetes can damage your blood vessels and the nerves that control your heart and blood vessels.

> High blood glucose from diabetes can damage your blood vessels and the nerves that control your heart and blood vessels.

The longer you have diabetes, the higher the chances that you will develop heart disease (1,2).

"People with diabetes tend to develop heart disease at a younger age than people without diabetes. In adults with diabetes, the most common causes of death are heart disease and stroke. Adults with diabetes are nearly twice as likely to die from heart disease or stroke as people without diabetes" (1,3).

1. U.S. Department of Health and Human Services. (n.d.). Diabetes, Heart Disease, and Stroke. Retrieved May 29, 2017, from https://www.niddk.nih.gov/health-information/diabetes/overview/preventing-problems/heart-disease-stroke

2. Huo, X. et al. (2016). Risk of non-fatal cardiovascular diseases in early-onset versus late-onset type 2 diabetes in China: a cross-sectional study. *The Lancet Diabetes & Endocrinology,* 4(2), 115-124.

3. National Centers for Disease Control and Prevention. National diabetes statistics report, 2014. https://www.cdc.gov/diabetes/pubs/statsreport14/national-diabetes-report-web.pdf. Accessed December 22, 2016.

Does obesity cause cancer?

Obesity is a known risk factor for at least 3 types of cancers, including breast, colorectal and pancreatic. North America has the highest rate of cancers caused by obesity. Almost 10 percent of cancer diagnoses among women were linked to obesity. According to the American Society of Clinical Oncology, "obesity may soon replace tobacco use as the leading preventable cause of cancer." About 33 percent of American adults are obese, and about 18 percent of adults smoke (1). In the past 25 years, obesity in the United States has increased while tobacco use has fallen.

According to The Cancer Treatment Centers of America, there are several factors in the relationship between obesity and cancer (1):

- "The hormone insulin-like growth factor, IGF-1, stimulates cell growth in obese people at possibly at twice the rate of normal-weight people, which may promote tumor growth.

- People who are obese have higher amounts of the hormone leptin, which appears to promote cell proliferation, and less of the hormone adiponectin, which may prevent cell growth.

- Fat tissue produces high levels of the hormone estrogen, which has been associated with the risk of breast and uterine cancers.

- Fat cells may affect other tumor growth regulators, such as mammalian target of rapamycin (mTOR) and AMP-activated protein kinase.

- People who are obese often have chronic low-level inflammation, which has been associated with increased cancer risk.

- Microbes that live in the gut of obese people activate bacteria to secrete chemicals that damage DNA and lead to tumor growth."

1. Cancer Treatment Centers of America. (2015, March 10). More new cancer cases linked to obesity. Retrieved from http://www.cancercenter.com/discussions/blog/more-new-cancer-cases-linked-to-obesity/?source=GGLPS01&channel=paid search&invsrc=Non_Branded_Paid_Search_Google_General_Search&utm_device=

c&utm_budget=Corporate&utm_site=GOOGLE
&utm_campaign=Non Brand%3ECancer%3E
General&utm_adgroup=Risk Factors%3EObesity
%3EPhrase&utm_term=obesity and cancer&utm_
matchtype=p&k_clickid=83a79a81-bbc1-4b9e-8c81-
f03578774302&k_profid=422&k_kwid=4136314

How type 2 diabetes relates to cancer

A strong and consistent increased risk of cancer is associated with type 2 diabetes. The strength of association depends on the cancer. The strongest relationships have been demonstrated for liver and pancreatic cancers. Reverse causality is likely one of the factors involved because the cancer itself can facilitate the onset of diabetes. "Risk of endometrial cancer appears to be doubled in women with diabetes. Risks of breast, colorectal, bladder, non-Hodgkin lymphoma (NHL) and kidney cancers are about 20–40% higher in people with type 2 diabetes" (1).

There are several hypothesized mechanisms for the association between diabetes and cancer, including insulin resistance and hyperinsulinemia (overproduction of insulin). Type 2 diabetes is characterized in the early stages by insulin resistance and consequent hyperinsulinemia. Hyperinsulinemia promotes tumor cell growth directly via insulin receptors (1). Overadministration of insulin as a treatment can also contribute to these effects, reinforcing the importance of prevention and reversal over treatment.

1. Johnson, J. et al. (2012). Diabetes and cancer (1): evaluating the temporal relationship between type 2 diabetes and cancer incidence. Diabetologia,55(6), 1607-1618. doi:10.1007/s00125-012-2525-1

Is Alzheimer's related to diabetes?

Alzheimer's is a chronic diet-related disease that results in dementia. Alzheimer's disease has been nicknamed "Type 3 diabetes." Diabetes is linked to Alzheimer's through insulin resistance and is one of the major factors that starts the brain-damage cascade. This damage impacts the memory of over half of people in their 80s. "More recent studies show people with diabetes have a four-fold greater risk for developing Alzheimer's. People with pre-diabetes or metabolic syndrome have an increased risk for having pre-dementia or mild cognitive impairment (MCI)" (1).

Eating sugar and refined carbs can cause pre-dementia and dementia. Removing sugar and refined carbs from the diet and adding significant quantities of healthy fat can prevent, and even reverse, pre-dementia and early dementia. Dr. Mark Hyman has observed improved memory, mood, and well-being in people engaged in the following programs:

- The Blood Sugar Solution
- The 10-Day Detox Diet
- Eat Fat, Get Thin

1. Hyman, M. (2016, February 12). Alzheimer's = Type 3 Diabetes [Web log post]. Retrieved from http://drhyman.com/blog/2016/02/12/ why-alzheimers-is-now-considered-type-3-diabetes/

How many people have Alzheimer's?

Dementia is a general term for loss of memory and other intellectual abilities serious enough to interfere with daily life.

The US ranks second globally for Alzheimer's death rates.

Alzheimer's disease accounts for 60 to 80 percent of dementia cases (1). The prevalence is related to the standard American diet—which is high in sugar and processed carbs and low in fat.

Alzheimer's doubles every 10 years after age 65. The Alzheimer's prevalence breakdown is as follows:

- 10 percent of 65-year-olds
- 25 percent of 75-year-olds
- 50 percent of 85-year-olds

The fastest growing segment of the American population is 85-year-olds. "Researchers predict Alzheimer's will affect 106 million people by 2050. It's now the seventh leading cause of death" (2). The US ranks second globally for Alzheimer's death rates. (3)

1. What Is Alzheimer's? (n.d.). Retrieved June 10, 2017, from http://www.alz.org/alzheimers_disease_what_is_alzheimers.asp

2. Hyman, M. (2016, February 12). Alzheimer's = Type 3 Diabetes [Web log post]. Retrieved from http://drhyman.com/blog/2016/02/12/why-alzheimers-is-now-considered-type-3-diabetes/

3. World Health Rankings. (n.d.). Retrieved June 10, 2017, from 3. http://www.worldlifeexpectancy.com/cause-of-death/alzheimers-dementia/by-country/

Can hypertension damage your body without signs or symptoms?

Most chronic diseases are silent in the beginning, having no signs or symptoms. This is one of the main reasons why people knowingly continue in unhealthy lifestyles in spite of the

eventual consequences. Hypertension is one of these conditions. Primary (essential) hypertension develops gradually over
many years, and it affects nearly everyone eventually. Most
people with high blood pressure have no signs or symptoms,
even if blood pressure reaches dangerous levels. According
to the Mayo Clinic, "Even without symptoms, damage to
blood vessels and your heart continues and can be detected.
Uncontrolled high blood pressure increases your risk of serious
health problems, including heart attack and stroke" (1). The
excessive pressure on your artery walls caused by high blood
pressure can damage your blood vessels as well as organs in
your body. The higher your blood pressure and the longer it
goes uncontrolled, the greater the damage.

The relationship between diabetes and hypertension is important because both contribute to blood vessel damage, and their
combined effects are greater than either one alone. This relationship is also important because blood vessel damage can
impact the entire body. Since it is common for diabetes and
hypertension to occur together, the combined effects will put
diabetics at greater risk for complications in their feet, eyes,
kidneys, and other parts of the body.

Uncontrolled high blood pressure can lead to (1):

- Heart attack or stroke. High blood pressure can
  cause hardening and thickening of the arteries
  (atherosclerosis), which can lead to a heart attack,
  stroke, or other complications.

- Aneurysm. Increased blood pressure can cause
  your blood vessels to weaken and bulge, forming
  an aneurysm. If an aneurysm ruptures, it can be
  life-threatening.

- Heart failure. To pump blood against the higher pressure in your vessels, your heart muscle thickens. Eventually, the thickened muscle may have a hard time pumping enough blood to meet your body's needs, which can lead to heart failure.

- Weakened and narrowed blood vessels in your kidneys. This can prevent these organs from functioning normally.

- Thickened, narrowed, or torn blood vessels in the eyes. This can result in vision loss.

- Metabolic syndrome. This syndrome is a cluster of disorders of your body's metabolism, including increased waist circumference; high triglycerides; low high-density lipoprotein (HDL) cholesterol, the "good" cholesterol; high blood pressure; and high insulin levels. These conditions make you more likely to develop diabetes, heart disease, and stroke.

- Trouble with memory or understanding. Uncontrolled high blood pressure may also affect your ability to think, remember, and learn. Trouble with memory or understanding concepts is more common in people with high blood pressure.

Many factors lead to the development of hypertension, including factors within our control and those outside of our control. Factors outside of our control include age, family history, and race. Factors within our control include smoking, diet, physical activity, stress, and the development of lifestyle-related chronic disease.

1. Mayo Foundation for Medical Education and Research. (2016, September 9). High blood pressure (hypertension). Retrieved May 29, 2017, from http://www.mayoclinic.org/

diseases-conditions/high-blood-pressure/basics/risk-factors/
con-20019580

How type 2 diabetes relates to hypertension and kidney disease

According to the American Heart Association, "Diabetes mellitus and hypertension are interrelated diseases that strongly predispose an individual to atherosclerotic cardiovascular disease" (1). High blood pressure frequency in individuals with diabetes doubles. Both conditions are dependent on lifestyle and genetic factors to varying degrees. "The prevalence of coexisting hypertension and diabetes appears to be increasing in industrialized nations" as their populations age (1).

What other complication are related to hypertension in diabetics? It is estimated that 35% to 75% of diabetic cardiovascular and renal complications can be attributed to hypertension. Hypertension often contributes to the development of nephropathy (kidney disease) in many diabetic individuals (2). Diabetic nephropathy occurs after 15 years of diabetes in 20% of those with type 2 diabetes (1). Nephropathy, in turn, is an important contributing factor to the development of hypertension. Small blood vessels are abundant in the kidneys because they help carry out the kidney's main function of filtering the blood. Diabetes damages small blood vessels throughout the body.

1. Sowers, J., & Epstein, M. (1995). Diabetes Mellitus and Associated Hypertension, Vascular Disease, and Nephropathy. Hypertension,26, 869-879. doi:10.1161/01.HYP.26.6.869

2. Mogensen, C. (1990). Prevention and treatment of renal disease in insulin-dependent diabetes mellitus. *Seminars in Nephrology,10*(3), 260-273.

Why does obesity increase your blood pressure?

As weight is gained, tissues are added to the body. The new tissues require more blood in order to supply oxygen and nutrients that the tissues need in order to survive. Increases in the volume of blood circulated through your blood vessels increase the pressure on your artery walls (1). This contributes to the increased risk of heart failure in obese people.

Losing weight achieves the opposite outcome. Fat tissue is lost as people lose weight, leading to a corresponding reduction in blood pressure. According to the National Institutes of Health, "losing even 10 pounds can lower your blood pressure—and losing weight has the biggest effect on those who are overweight and already have hypertension" (2).

Inactivity contributes to hypertension. People who are physically inactive tend to have higher heart rates. Higher heart rates require your heart to work harder. Higher heart rates also increase the force on your arteries (1). Insufficient physical activity also increases the risk of being overweight. Excess weight further complicates health issues because it is involved in all of the major chronic diseases (3).

1. Mayo Clinic. (2016, September 9). Diseases and Conditions High blood pressure (hypertension). Retrieved from http://www.mayoclinic.org/diseases-conditions/high-blood-pressure/basics/risk-factors/con-20019580

2. National Institutes of Health. (n.d.). Your Guide to Lowering Blood Pressure. Retrieved May 29, 2017, from https://www.nhlbi.nih.gov/files/docs/public/heart/hbp_low.pdf

3. National Center for Health Statistics. (n.d.). Deaths and Mortality. Retrieved May 29, 2017, from https://www.cdc.gov/nchs/fastats/deaths.htm

How does chronic disease impact stress?

The number and type of chronic diseases a person has affects stress levels. Many people have multiple chronic diseases such as diabetes, heart disease, obesity, and cancer. All of these can occur simultaneously. Stress levels increase with the number of chronic diseases. Multiple chronic diseases leads to increased medical costs, decreased capacity for life and work, and decreased quality of life. All of these factors increase stress. By increasing stress, chronic conditions also increase the risk of high blood pressure in the following ways (1):

- Chronic disease causes stress directly at the physiological level.

- Chronic disease causes stress at the psychological level from concerns about the implications of the disease for financial, relational, and physical health.

- Unhealthy coping mechanisms further complicate the situation. If people try to reduce stress by eating, tobacco use, or alcohol consumption, the problems associated with high blood pressure may increase.

- The number and type of chronic diseases a person has also affects stress levels. Many people have multiple chronic diseases such as diabetes, heart disease, obesity, and cancer. All of these can occur simultaneously. As the number of chronic diseases increases, so does stress level.

- Stress can play a role in the following chronic conditions (2):
  - headaches
  - high blood pressure
  - heart problems
  - diabetes

- ○ skin conditions
- ○ asthma
- ○ arthritis
- ○ depression
- ○ anxiety

According to a Web MD, "The Occupational Safety and Health Administration (OSHA) declared stress a hazard of the workplace. Stress costs American industry more than $300 billion annually" (2). The U.S. has low rankings for stress related conditions compared to other countries (3). 86% of other countries ranked higher in managing stress. This is a significant result because 90% of all doctors visits are for stress-related ailments (2). Stress and chronic disease reinforce each other. Stress especially impacts T2D and obesity because it drives cravings for comfort food.

> 90% of all doctor visits are for stress-related ailments.

1. Mayo Clinic. (2016, September 9). Diseases and Conditions High blood pressure (hypertension). Retrieved from http://www.mayoclinic.org/diseases-conditions/high-blood-pressure/basics/risk-factors/con-20019580

2. Web MD (n.d.). The Effects of Stress on Your Body. Retrieved May 29, 2017, from http://www.webmd.com/balance/stress-management/effects-of-stress-on-your-body

3. World Economic Forum. (2013). The Human Capital Report (Rep.).

Diet and autoimmune disease

According to researchers, autoimmune diseases such as multiple sclerosis (MS), rheumatoid arthritis (RA), inflammatory bowel disease (IBD), type 1 diabetes (T1D), and psoriasis (Ps) share common hallmarks, including involvement of T cell-mediated autoimmune mechanisms and a chronic disease condition that often requires life-long disease management. A relatively low rate of autoimmune disease onset between identical twins suggests environmental factors, including diet, as important triggers of disease (1).

For example, the incidence of multiple sclerosis (MS) may be positively associated with the consumption of milk, animal fat, and meat as well as total energy intake and obesity. Diet can also decrease MS risk if it contains high amounts of certain polyunsaturated fatty acids and plant fiber. Other studies found beneficial effects of fish oils, vegetables, and fresh fruits. The linkage to diet was also suggested by studies involving rheumatoid arthritis (RA). These epidemiological findings in MS and RA were not corroborated by the majority of more recent case-controlled studies. The inconclusive results of epidemiologic studies do not justify omitting nutrients as influential factors, but rather highlight the challenge of detecting diet effects in heterogeneous populations (non-twin studies). "Subjects prone to autoimmunity have complex individual risk profiles comprised of genetic and environmental determinants that make their response to nutritional cues diverse" (1).

1.   Manzel, A. et al. (2014). Role of "Western Diet" in Inflammatory Autoimmune Diseases. Curr Allergy Asthma Rep.,14(1), 404. doi:10.1007/ s11882-013-0404-6

How the Western diet relates to autoimmunity

High-carb diets stimulate fat storage in white adipose tissue (WAT) through the storage hormone insulin. White adipose tissue leads to systemic inflammation because WAT is not an inert tissue. "It is regarded an 'endocrine organ' releasing a large variety of pro-inflammatory molecules such as TNF-α, IL-6, leptin, resistin, and C-reactive protein" (1). These molecules ("adipokines") account for a chronic low-grade systemic inflammation in obese subjects. Chronic inflammatory signals can have a profound impact on T immune cell populations, and it has been shown that diet-induced obesity can promote a TH17-biased immunity in humans (1).

"Th17 and IL-17 immune cells play important roles in the clearance of extracellular bacterial and fungal infections."Strong evidence implicates the Th17 cells in several autoimmune disorders including type I diabetes, multiple sclerosis, psoriasis, rheumatoid arthritis, inflammatory bowel disease, systemic lupus erythematosus, and asthma" (2)

1. Manzel, A. et al. (2014). Role of "Western Diet" in Inflammatory Autoimmune Diseases. Curr Allergy Asthma Rep.,14(1), 404. doi:10.1007/s11882-013-0404-6

2. Kennedy Bedoya, S. et al. (2013). Th17 Cells in Immunity and Autoimmunity. Clinical and Developmental Immunology,2013. doi:10.1155/2013/986789

5

CHRONIC DISEASE REVERSAL

Reverse diabetes/ Reverse a set of chronic diseases

THERE IS A growing body of evidence that most of our chronic diseases in America are diet-driven. This means that diet can also be used reverse these conditions. The chances of reversal depend on several factors, but there is good news for everyone. According to Dr. Mike Roizen of the Cleveland Clinic, 98% of people can pull plaque out of their arteries to some degree through healthy diet and lifestyle. (1) Prevention of some diet-driven chronic diseases is a virtual certainty if healthy lifestyle begins early and is maintained.

The central dietary components of diet driven diseases such as diabetes, cancer, Alzheimer's disease, heart disease, and obesity are simple carbohydrates and sweeteners. The disease most directly linked to these foods is type 2 diabetes. More and more people are reversing diabetes by replacing simple carbohydrates with non-starchy veggies and healthy fats such as olive oil and coconut oil. As they reverse diabetes, doctors are finding other chronic diseases reverse such as heart disease, cancer, obesity, and Alzheimer's. According to Dr. Mark Hyman of the Cleveland Clinic, "Diabesity (a broader term that includes diabetes associated conditions) is the underlying cause of most heart disease, cancer, and premature death in the world" (2).

Just as chronic disease screening can be simplified through diabetes and obesity, the central components of the disease, the reversal of chronic disease can also be simplified through diabetes and obesity. Reversal of type 2 diabetes and obesity can facilitate reversal of heart disease and, to a lesser extent, cancer, Alzheimer's, and some autoimmune diseases. Doctors in functional medicine and other medical disciplines have reported reversal results in each of these cases. Chronic diseases previously thought not amenable to prevention have been found to be highly preventable.

1. The impact of wellness on community sustainability [Interview by T. Schierer]. (2016, November). JETT Radio interview with Dr. Mike Roizen https://vimeo.com/193400128

2. Hyman, M. (2014, December 18). 7 Steps to Reverse Obesity and Diabetes [Web log post]. Retrieved from http://drhyman.com/blog/2014/12/18/7-ways-reverse-obesity-diabetes/

New research is needed to maximize chronic disease reversal

Because we know that the removal of sugar and simple carbohydrates from the diet effectively facilitates reversal of pre-diabetes and early-stage diabetes, studies are needed that compare reversal rates amongst different types of diets and preventive health care regimes. This is needed because:

- Different people metabolize food differently
- Different people have different food sensitivities
- There are subtypes of type 2 diabetes that probably respond differently to exercise (1)
- Different people have different genetic susceptibility to acquiring diabetes and other chronic diseases
- The duration of the diabetic state impacts the ease of reversal
- The age of diabetes onset has an impact on ease of reversal
- The current level of health has an impact on the ease of reversal

1. Spero, D. (2016, March 9). What Kind of Type 2 Diabetes Do You Have? [Web log post]. Retrieved from https://www.diabetesselfmanagement.com/blog/kind-type-2-diabetes/

Reverse diabetes/ reverse obesity

Two of the most strongly related reversible chronic diseases are diabetes and obesity. Morbidly obese patients can reverse type 2 diabetes within a few weeks of getting a gastric bypass surgery, even if they haven't lost that much weight. When disease-producing food is removed and replaced with healthy food, healing happens quickly. Dr. Mark Hyman had a patient lose 45 pounds and get off 54 units of insulin and all his diabetes medications (1).

These diet-related conditions reinforce in both directions: acquisition and reversal. Obesity probably comes first in most cases. Both are caused by poor diet and lifestyle habits. One disease does not reverse the other. Both are reversed by healthy diet and lifestyle. This reversal can occur without drugs and surgery. Moreover, fewer medications correlate with better health: the opposite of the belief that medication is needed to stay healthy.

1. Hyman, M. (2014, December 18). 7 Steps to Reverse Obesity and Diabetes [Web log post]. Retrieved from http://drhyman.com/blog/2014/12/1 8/7-ways-reverse-obesity-diabetes/

Are the steps to reverse obesity the same as the steps to diabetes reversal?

According to Dr. Hyman, the steps to reverse diabetes and obesity are as follows:

Remove or replace simple carbohydrates: High carb consumption creates high insulin levels, eventually leading to insulin resistance and Type 2 diabetes. The most important factor in reducing the risk of type 2 diabetes and obesity or reversing their impact is to eliminate or dramatically reduce sugar in all its many forms (1).

Exercise: There is a wide range of exercise regimes that improve health. Vigorous exercise is the key to balancing blood sugar and lowering insulin levels (heart rate up to 70–80% of its maximum capacity for 60 minutes, up to six times a week).

Sufficient sleep: Sleep deprivation damages your metabolism, spikes sugar and carb cravings, and increases your risk for numerous diseases including Type 2 diabetes. One study among healthy subjects found even a partial night's poor sleep could induce insulin resistance. That's why you must prioritize sleep so you get eight hours of solid, uninterrupted shuteye every night.

Control stress levels: Stress increases levels of insulin, cortisol, and inflammatory compounds called cytokines. This drives the metabolic dysfunction that leads to weight gain, insulin resistance, and eventually Type 2 diabetes.

Measure to improve: Research demonstrates that people who track their results lose twice as much weight. Track what you eat, your weight, waist size, body mass index (BMI), and blood pressure (optional). Many patients become inspired by seeing improvement.

1. Hyman, M. (2014, December 18). 7 Steps to Reverse Obesity and Diabetes [Web log post]. Retrieved from http://drhyman.com/blog/2014/12/18/7-ways-reverse-obesity-diabetes/

Reverse diabetes/ Reverse heart disease

Dean Ornish, MD, is founder and president of the Preventive Medicine Research Institute and Clinical Professor of Medicine, University of California, San Francisco. He has written six best-selling books, including Dr. Dean Ornish's Program for Reversing Heart Disease. One of the most important aspects of his disease reversal work was direct measurement of the heart disease reversal process. "Within a year on our program, even severely blocked arteries in the heart became less blocked, and there was even more reversal after 5 years.

That's compared with other patients in our study, in which the heart just got worse and worse" (1).

Ornish had patients with the worst possible damage, those needing a heart transplant, enroll in his reversal program while waiting for a transplant. Some of them improved to the point of no longer needing a transplant. "Our studies show that with significant lifestyle changes, blood flow to the heart and its ability to pump normally improve in less than a month, and the frequency of chest pains fell by 90% in that time" (1). His team also reported that 82% of experimental-group patients had an average change towards heart disease regression. Comprehensive lifestyle changes may be able to bring about regression of even severe coronary atherosclerosis after only 1 year, without the use of lipid-lowering drugs (2).

Under the Ornish Reversal Diet, only 10% of your diet comes from fat; 15–20% comes from protein, and 70–75% comes from complex carbohydrates. Even though this low-fat approach differs significantly from functional medicine, the common element among reversal diets is the 70% plus level of whole, non-starchy, plant-based foods. Functional medicine diets also recommend 75% veggies, including unlimited amounts of cruciferous vegetables (broccoli, cauliflower, brussel sprouts) (3). An additional consideration is that the holistic nature of the Ornish program, which included stress management and non-physical health, may have been as important to the reversal results as the diet (4).

Since diabetes is the most prevalent diet-driven chronic disease, it would be logical to use a diet fine-tuned to diabetes reversal as a standard base diet. Adoption of a diabetes reversal diet as a national standard diet would essentially begin a nationwide prevention and reversal of all chronic, diet-driven diseases, eventually saving us trillions of dollars in healthcare and other aspects of the economy. Standard diets created our epidemics of diabetes, heart disease, Alzheimer's, and other chronic diseases. Why not reverse these epidemics with a standard diet?

Dr. Caldwell B. Esselstyn, Jr., Preventive Medicine Consultant, Cleveland Clinic also reported significant heart disease reversal results. In his 21-year Cleveland Clinic nutritional study (5), he reversed advanced coronary artery disease in patients who had already undergone bypasses and angioplasties; "some had even been told by their cardiologist that they had less than a year to live" (6). Those patients told by expert cardiologists 20 years ago that they had less than a year to live remained alive (6).

Compliant patients' angina diminished and largely disappeared. They achieved and maintained cholesterol goals: to maintain a total cholesterol less than 150 mg/dL and an LDL-cholesterol less than 80 mg/dL through plant-based nutrition. At this cholesterol level, the body does not deposit fat and cholesterol into arteries. Angiographic evidence showed their disease had selectively reversed. Most importantly, Dr. Esselstyn discovered that patients are empowered when they know they can control their disease, rather than rely on risky, expensive, inconsistent drugs, stents, or bypasses.

According to Dr. Esselstyn, plant-based nutrition can eliminate some diseases. The long-term study was built on epidemiological evidence in plant-based cultures, such as rural China, the Papua Highlanders, central Africa, and the Tarahumara Indians, where the inhabitants are virtually free of coronary disease.

> Heart disease patients told that they had less than a year to live remained alive 20 years later.

1. Shaw, G. (n.d.). Can You Reverse Heart Disease? Retrieved May 29, 2017, from http://www.webmd.com/heart-disease/features/can-you-reverse-heart-disease#1

2. Ornish, D. (1990). Can lifestyle changes reverse coronary heart disease? The Lifestyle Heart Trial. Lancet,336(8708), 129-133. Retrieved from https://www.ncbi.nlm.nih.gov/pubmed/1973470.

3. Hyman, M. (2016, March 30). Fat: What I Got Wrong, What I Got Right [Web log post]. Retrieved from http://drhyman.com/blog/2016/03/30/fat-what-i-got-wrong-what-i-got-right/

4. Teicholz, N. (2014). Big Fat Surprise. New York, NY: Simon and Shuster, Chapter 7

5. Esselstyn, C. B. (2007). Prevent and reverse heart disease. New York, NY: Penguin Group.

6. Esselstyn, C., Jr. (2007). We Can Prevent and Even Reverse Coronary Artery Heart Disease. MedGenMed,9(3), 46. Retrieved from https://www.ncbi.nlm.nih.gov/pmc/articles/PMC2100124/.

Reverse diabetes/ reverse cancer

Cancer is a chronic disease linked to toxins, smoking, diet, and stress. Insulin resistance, prediabetes, and type 2 diabetes dramatically increase the risk of most common cancers such as prostate, breast, colon, pancreas, and liver (1). It turns out that cancer cells feed on sugar and have a high concentration of insulin growth factor receptors. The diabetic environment promotes cancer cell growth (2).

> Cancer cells feed on sugar.

Cancer is a diet-driven disease. Bad diets can lead to cancer, and good diets can help reverse cancer. Vegetables and fruits contain powerful anti-cancer compounds. People with the highest consumption of broccoli and other cruciferous vegetables had the lowest risk of cancer (1). Omega-3 fats also have anti-cancer properties because they reduce inflammation and improve insulin resistance.

1. Hyman, M. (2016). Eat fat, get thin: why the fat we eat is the key to sustained weight loss and vibrant health. New York: Little, Brown and Company. p. 167-168

2. Taubes, G. (2017). The case against sugar. New York: Alfred A. Knopf. Ch 14

Reverse diabetes/ reverse Alzheimer's

Coconut is mainly grown in the tropics for its nutritional and medicinal values. Coconut oil contains high levels of saturated fat composed mainly of medium-chain fatty acids (MCFA). Coconut is classified as a highly nutritious 'functional food.' It is rich in dietary fiber, vitamins, and minerals. MCFAs are easily absorbed and metabolized by the liver and can be converted to ketones. "Ketone bodies are an important alternative energy source in the brain, and may be beneficial to people developing or already with memory impairment, as in Alzheimer's disease (AD)" (1).

In addition to Alzheimer's, coconut may be beneficial in the treatment of obesity, dyslipidemia, elevated LDL, insulin resistance, and hypertension. All these are risk factors for cardiovascular disease, type 2 diabetes, and AD. Coconut contains phenolic compounds and hormones (cytokinins) which may assist in preventing the aggregation of amyloid-β peptide. Aggregation of amyloid-β peptide is a key step in the pathogenesis of AD. Several studies have explored the potential role of coconut supplementation as a therapeutic option in the prevention and management of AD (1). Many thought that

Alzheimer's is irreversible, but functional medicine doctors are documenting cases of Alzheimer's reversal (2)

Diabetes reversal diets recommend the use and direct consumption of coconut oil (2). In addition, diabetics have reported beneficial outcomes from ketogenic (high-fat) diets including coconut oil. Diabetes reversal diets and programs are compatible with reversal of Alzheimer's disease but may have their greatest effect in the prevention of Alzheimer's. The underlying causes of Alzheimer's disease begin with high blood sugar. The cycle starts when we over-consume sugar and under-consume fat, which leads to diabesity. Diabesity leads to inflammation, and inflammation damages the brain (2). Dementia and cognitive decline can be reversed. Balancing insulin and blood sugar levels allows you to overcome diabesity; it balances your mood, helps your focus, helps boost your energy level, and prevents all of the age-related brain diseases, including Alzheimer's (2).

1. Fernando, W. M. et al. (2015). The role of dietary coconut for the prevention and treatment of Alzheimer's disease: potential mechanisms of action. Br J Nutr.,114(1), 1-14. doi:10.1017/S0007114515001452

2. Hyman, M. (2016, February 12). Alzheimer's = Type 3 Diabetes [Web log post]. Retrieved from http://drhyman.com/blog/2016/02/12/why-alzheimers-is-now-considered-type-3-diabetes/

Reversal rates can guide the way

> Disease reversal rates can organize and focus future medical science.

Millions of different experiments have been conducted in the history of science. They are guided by a desire for higher level understanding of biological function or to find solutions for problems. Disease reversal rates can organize and focus future medical science. If disease parameters are known, and the disease is reversible, then its reversal can be tracked.

Reversal rates can result in the establishment of:

- Approved or recommended preventative health care (PHC) regimes for specific diseases
- A list of the most effective diets for specific diseases
- A list of diseases most amenable to prevention
- A list of diseases most amenable to reversal
- A reversal timetable for specific diseases
- A list of co-reversal rates for some co-morbidities (e.g., Type 2 diabetes and heart disease co-reversal)
- A list of co-morbidities that will improve with specific PHC regimes
- A list of exercise regimes or characteristics that maximize reversal for specific diseases
- Identification of transition points from treatment to PHC
- Healthcare cost savings estimates

PART 2

THE REVERSAL PROCESS FOR TYPE 2 DIABETES

6
WHAT IS DIABETES?

DIABETES IS A progressive disease in which a combination of insulin resistance in muscle, liver, and fat cells and failure of pancreatic beta cell function lead to a loss of glycemic control. Some people can consistently make more insulin in response to increased sugar intake. Diabetics cannot. In type 2 diabetes, cells do not adapt to impaired glucose tolerance. This failure appears to be related to a reduction in insulin secretion as well as a reduction in the total number of islets cells that produce insulin (1). According to the Diabetes Research Institute Foundation, "Islets actually are clusters of cells in the pancreas. "Within each islet are several types of cells, which work together to regulate blood sugar. One cell type is the beta cell. Beta cells sense sugar in the blood and release the necessary amount of insulin to maintain normal blood sugar levels. The loss of these cells means the body can no longer produce insulin, the hormone required to convert food into energy for the body's cells" (2).

1. Bray, George et. al. "Prediabetes & Insulin Resistance." National Institute of Diabetes and Digestive and Kidney Diseases. Retrieved 22 June 2017, from http://diabetes. niddk.nih.gov/dm/pubs/insulinresistance/#resistance

2. "What are Islet Cells?" Diabetes Research Institute Foundation. N.p., n.d. Web. 22 June 2017.

Question: How would you define diabetes?

Realities of a diabetic disease state

When used as a medication, insulin does not completely abolish the progressive loss of pancreatic beta cell function and can have harmful effects. Its use is also associated with hypoglycemia and weight gain (1). If T2D progresses to the point of requiring treatment, the following changes ensue if preventative lifestyle adjustments are not made:

> Pancreatic beta cell decline can occur 12 years before diagnosis, and it continues throughout the disease process.

Abnormal beta cell volume and number: Subjects with impaired fasting glucose had a decreased number of beta cells and a decreased relative beta cell volume, suggesting that this is an early process and mechanistically important in the development of type 2 diabetes. Thus, damage to the pancreas is occurring before the onset of diabetes. Ultimately, the pancreas "declines in size" as T2D progresses (1).

Loss of beta cell function: Progressive loss of beta cell function and reduced beta cell mass lead to worsening glycemic control and development of complications. Beta cell decline can begin 12 years or more before diagnosis, and it continues throughout the disease process. It is well advanced by the time a person's plasma glucose level is in the diabetic range. The beta cells in the pancreas try to keep up with this increased demand for insulin by producing more. As long as the beta cells are able to produce enough insulin to overcome the insulin resistance, blood glucose levels stay in the healthy range (2). As the loss of glycemic control progresses, so does the loss of beta cell function. Chronic hyperglycemia depletes insulin secretory granules from beta cells, lessening the amount of insulin available to be released in response to new glucose intake. The exact mechanisms responsible for impaired beta cell function have yet to be elucidated at the molecular level.

Beta cells of diabetics produce less insulin: Insulin secretion from islets of organ donors who had diabetes was significantly less than that of control subjects, and islet yield decreased as disease duration lengthened (2).

Repeated and vigorous intervention: Patients with diabetes require repeated and vigorous treatment intervention. Even with most therapies, A1C will increase by 1% every 2 years (1). Thus, pancreatic function decreases even with treatment for those progressing to a diabetic state.

Progressive loss of glycemic control: Failure to implement healthy lifestyle interventions results in worsening glucose control, eventually resulting in perpetuating circle of hyperglycemia and glucose toxicity.

Cellular failure in late stages of diabetes (1): In late stages of T2D, the progressive rise in the insulin resistance exacerbates beta cell failure. Beta cell failure includes permanent loss of cell

> Beta cell failure includes permanent loss of cell function and cell death. Both are serious complications of the disease that ultimately contribute to early death.

function and cell death. Both are serious complications of the disease that ultimately contribute to early death.

1. Fonseca, V. A. (2009). Defining and Characterizing the Progression of Type 2 Diabetes. Diabetes Care. 32(2), 5151-5156. doi:10.2337/dc09-S301

2. Bray, G. et. al. "Prediabetes & Insulin Resistance." National Institute of Diabetes and Digestive and Kidney Diseases. Retrieved 22 June 2017, from http://diabetes.niddk.nih.gov/dm/pubs/insulinresistance/#resistance.

Question: What are some of the advantages of preventing type 2 diabetes?

Question: What are some advantages of getting off insulin?

Insulin resistance: In an insulin resistant state, muscle, fat, and liver cells do not respond properly to insulin and thus cannot easily absorb glucose from the bloodstream. As a result, the body needs higher levels of insulin to help glucose enter cells (1). Pancreatic beta cells normally respond to insulin resistance by increasing their output of insulin to meet the needs of tissues. Development of type 2 diabetes essentially stems from a failure of the beta cells to adequately compensate for insulin resistance. Some obese individuals do not progress to diabetes because their beta cells continue to function adequately to cope with insulin resistance by increasing insulin secretion.

1. Bray, G. et al. (n.d.). Prediabetes & Insulin Resistance. Retrieved June 22, 2017, from https://www.niddk.nih.gov/health-information/diabetes/overview/what-is-diabetes/prediabetes-insulin-resistance#resistance

Diabetes-related health conditions

There are multiple reasons why maintaining a healthy weight is worth the effort not least of which includes avoiding serious complications associated with T2D.

The rate of heart attack, stroke, and cardiovascular death was about twice as high in diabetics as in non-diabetics. The following conditions related to T2D were reported by the American Diabetes Association (1).

> The rate of heart attack, stroke, and cardiovascular death was about twice as high in diabetics as in non-diabetics.

Hypoglycemia: In 2011, about 282,000 emergency room visits for adults aged 18 years or older had hypoglycemia as the first-listed diagnosis and diabetes as an additional diagnosis.

Hypertension: In 2009–2012, of adults aged 18 years or older with diagnosed diabetes, 71% had blood pressure greater than or equal to 140/90 millimeters of mercury or used prescription medications to lower high blood pressure.

Dyslipidemia: In 2009–2012, of adults aged 18 years or older with diagnosed diabetes, 65% had blood LDL cholesterol greater than or equal to 100 mg/dl or used cholesterol-lowering medications.

CVD Death Rates: In 2003–2006, after adjusting for population age differences, cardiovascular disease death rates were about 1.7 times higher among adults aged 18 years or older with diagnosed diabetes than among adults without diagnosed diabetes.

Heart Attack Rates: In 2010, after adjusting for population age differences, hospitalization rates for heart attack were 1.8 times higher among adults aged 20 years or older with diagnosed diabetes than among adults without diagnosed diabetes.

Stroke: In 2010, after adjusting for population age differences, hospitalization rates for stroke were 1.5 times higher among adults with diagnosed diabetes aged 20 years or older compared to those without diagnosed diabetes.

Blindness and Eye Problems: In 2005–2008, of adults with diabetes aged 40 years or older, 4.2 million (28.5%) people had diabetic retinopathy, damage to the small blood vessels in the retina that may result in loss of vision.

Kidney Disease: Diabetes was listed as the primary cause of kidney failure in 44% of all new cases in 2011.

- In 2011, 49,677 people of all ages began treatment for kidney failure due to diabetes.

- In 2011, a total of 228,924 people of all ages with kidney failure due to diabetes were living on chronic dialysis or with a kidney transplant.

Amputations: In 2010, about 73,000 non-traumatic lower-limb amputations were performed in adults aged 20 years or older with diagnosed diabetes.

About 60% of non-traumatic lower-limb amputations among people aged 20 years or older occur in people with diagnosed diabetes.

CDC summary of serious health complications associated with T2D (2)
Blindness
Kidney failure
Heart disease
Stroke
Amputation of toes, feet, or legs
Risk of death for people with diabetes is 50% greater

1. Statistics About Diabetes. (2017, April 05). Retrieved from http://www.diabetes.org/diabetes-basics/statistics/

2. A Snapshot: Diabetes in the United States. (n.d.). Retrieved June 22, 2017, from https://www.cdc.gov/media/DPK/2014/images/diabetes-report/Infographic1-web.pdf

Question: What concerns you most from the list of diabetes-related condition?

Type 2 diabetes pathogenesis

90% of pre-diabetics don't know it

By the late 1990s, an epidemic of type 2 diabetes had taken hold in the United States. The epidemic has spread throughout the world. It is tied to sugar consumption more than obesity. Lack of awareness has impacted this issue in very significant ways. The lack of awareness in the scientific community regarding differentiation of caloric quality and the value of healthy fats led to erroneous diet recommendations that greatly augmented the type 2 epidemic. Scientists and citizens all believed that all fat was bad and that all calories were created equal.

The need for individuals to regularly test their blood sugar is another area that lacked awareness. Over 90% of prediabetics are either unaware or unconcerned that they have pre-diabetes because it is asymptomatic. Blood sugar testing is an essential component to reversing the epidemic of type 2 diabetes. Diabetes education also plays an important role.

If you have friends, coworkers, and family who exhibit some of the risk factors for diabetes, ask them if they had their blood sugar tested. Inexpensive blood sugar meters are available at drugstores for as little as $10. The combination of faulty nutritional research and faulty nutritional recommendations in combination with the lack of testing has been a potent combination. The reverse approach should be able to counter or slow the progress of the epidemic. This reversal has begun. The nutritional research espousing healthy fats is emerging now. Two leaders in the field of chronic disease reversal published new books in 2016. Dr. Mark Hyman of the Cleveland Clinic published *Eat Fat, Get Thin,* and Dr. David Ludwig of Harvard University published *Always Hungry.*

How soon does diabetes damage the body?

People do not feel physical pain from prediabetics, but damage is occurring to the cells in the pancreas and throughout the body before blood sugar control is lost (1). "Prediabetes is associated with the simultaneous presence of insulin resistance and β-cell dysfunction. Observational evidence shows associations of prediabetes with early forms of nephropathy, chronic kidney disease, small fibre neuropathy, diabetic retinopathy, and increased risk of macrovascular disease" (2).

If damage is occurring to our bodies when we eat too much of the wrong kinds of foods, does it matter whether it is painless? Smoking is similar. It can be pain-free for decades while cellular damage is occurring. In time, it leads to massive end-stage pain as cancer takes over. Long-term health considerations lead to healthy choices. Healthy lifestyle is not just beneficial for the long-term. It has many benefits in the present, including energy level, mental clarity, and lower medical costs.

> Diabetes can be pain-free for decades while cellular damage is occurring.

1. Tabak, A. et al. (2012). Prediabetes: A high-risk state for developing diabetes. Lancet,379(9833), 2279-2290. doi:10.1016/S0140-6736(12)60283-9

Summary of insulin's role in blood glucose control

When blood glucose levels rise after a meal, the pancreas releases insulin into the blood. Insulin and glucose then travel in the blood to cells throughout the body. Insulin performs the following functions:

- Insulin helps muscle, fat, and liver cells absorb glucose from the bloodstream, lowering blood glucose levels.

- Insulin stimulates the liver and muscle tissue to store excess glucose.

- Insulin also lowers blood glucose levels by reducing glucose production in the liver.

In diabetics, insulin is not able to perform its function as well because cells throughout the body become resistant to insulin. This makes the pancreas work harder to overcome insulin resistance. "In insulin resistance, muscle, fat, and liver cells do not respond properly to insulin and thus cannot easily absorb glucose from the bloodstream. As a result, the body needs higher levels of insulin to help glucose enter cells. The beta cells in the pancreas try to keep up with this increased demand for insulin by producing more. As long as the beta cells are able to produce enough insulin to overcome the insulin resistance, blood glucose levels stay in the healthy range. Without enough insulin, excess glucose builds up in the bloodstream, leading to diabetes, prediabetes, and other serious health disorders" (1).

1. Bray, G. et al. (n.d.). Prediabetes & Insulin Resistance. Retrieved June 22, 2017, from https://www.niddk. nih.gov/health-information/diabetes/overview/ what-is-diabetes/prediabetes-insulin-resistance#resistance

How fast do pre-diabetics develop diabetes?

The case for preventative healthcare is strong. Diabetes is a particularly clear case because of its progressive nature and its preventability and reversibility. 95% of diabetes is preventable (type 2) and about 5% is not (type1). Type 2 diabetes is also reversible, and the sooner someone begins the reversal process through healthy lifestyle changes, the greater the chances of reversal. For type 2 diabetics, the chances of reversal decrease by 50% if reversal is started 8 years after diagnosis compared with up to an 80% chance of reversal within 4 years of diagnosis (1). Prediabetics convert to diabetes at the rate of 5–10% per year. (2) Without Lifestyle intervention, 50% of prediabetics could convert to diabetes within 5 to 10 years, and the entire group could convert to diabetes within 10 to 20 years.

> Prediabetics convert to diabetes at the rate of 5–10% per year.

It is difficult to imagine a stronger case for lifestyle intervention than diabetes. Yet people do not consider the long-term costs. Diabetes moves slowly, and people don't experience severe complications until the disease is very advanced. This advanced state takes years to develop and so do the diabetes associated diseases such as heart disease, kidney disease, and neuropathy. The conditions then combine to create very unpleasant, costly, and prolonged end of life stages all of which can be prevented. When considering whether prevention is worth it, a helpful question to ask is, "what will it cost me to not prevent?"

1. Steven, S., Lim, E., & Taylor, R. (2013). Treatment Population response to information on reversibility of Type 2 diabetes. *Diabet Med,30*(4), 135-138. doi: 10.1111/dme.12116

2. Tabak, A. et al. (2012). Prediabetes: A high-risk state for developing diabetes. Lancet,379(9833), 2279-2290. doi:10.1016/S0140-6736(12)60283-9

When should we suspect low blood sugar?

Have you experienced any of the following symptoms from the list below? Tests to determine insulin levels are most frequently ordered in response to low glucose and/or when someone has acute or chronic symptoms of low blood glucose (hypoglycemia). Symptoms of hypoglycemia may include (1):

- Sweating
- Palpitations
- Hunger
- Confusion
- Blurred vision
- Dizziness
- Fainting
- In serious cases, seizures, and loss of consciousness

What about the symptoms of high blood sugar? Symptoms of high blood sugar include (2):

- Severe thirst
- Frequent urination
- Unexplained weight loss
- Increased hunger
- Tingling in your hands or feet

1. The Test. (n.d.). Retrieved June 22, 2017, from https://labtestsonline.org/understanding/analytes/insulin/tab/test/
2. High Glucose: What It Means and How to Treat It. (n.d.). Retrieved June 22, 2017, from http://www.joslin.org/info/high_glucose_what_it_means_and_how_to_treat_it.html

How high blood sugar damages the body

According to Web MD (1), high blood sugar damages the body because:

- High sugar levels slowly erode the ability of cells in your pancreas to make insulin. The organ overcompensates, and insulin levels stay too high. Over time, the pancreas is permanently damaged.
- High levels of blood sugar can cause changes that lead to a hardening of the blood vessels or atherosclerosis.

Almost any part of your body can be harmed by too much sugar. Damaged blood vessels cause problems such as:

- Kidney disease or kidney failure, requiring dialysis
- Strokes

- Heart attacks
- Vision loss or blindness
- Weakened immune system, with a greater risk of infections
- Erectile dysfunction
- Nerve damage, also called neuropathy, that causes tingling, pain, or less sensation in your feet, legs, and hands
- Poor circulation to the legs and feet
- Slow wound-healing and the potential for amputation in rare cases
  1. High blood sugar, diabetes, and your body. (n.d.). Retrieved June 22, 2017, from http://www.webmd.com/diabetes/how-sugar-affects-diabetes#1

How T2D damages blood vessels

Researchers at Washington University in St. Louis studied "FASTie" mice that had been genetically engineered to understand how blood vessels become damaged in diabetes (1).

Molecular root defect: Researchers Xiaochao Wei and Clay F. Semenkovich, MD, discovered that fatty acid synthase (FAS) preferentially makes a lipid (palmitoylation) that allows nitric oxide synthase (NOS) to hook to the cell membrane and to produce normal, healthy blood vessels. This attachment to the cell membrane is essential to its function, and it is defective in diabetics.

Result of defective FAS: In the FASTie mice, blood vessels were leaky, and in cases when the vessel was injured, the mice were unable to generate new blood vessel growth. The mice were more susceptible to the consequences of infection similar to people with diabetes. The experimental mice couldn't repair cell damage that occurred (1).

Human model: In human endothelial cells, the palmitoylation deficiency link to diabetes suggests possible treatments of the vascular complications of diabetes. This may include several options that restore FAS function (1). "Free fatty acids are known to play a key role in promoting loss of insulin sensitivity in type 2 diabetes mellitus but the underlying mechanism is still unclear. It has been postulated that an increase in the intracellular concentration of fatty acid metabolites activates a serine kinase cascade, which leads to defects in insulin signaling downstream to the insulin receptor" (2).

In addition, the complex network of adipokines released from fat tissue modulates the response of tissues to insulin, including reduction in insulin receptor gene expression. Dysfunction of several molecules involved in the intracellular processing of the signal provided by insulin results in insulin resistance. These molecules are potential new targets for the treatment and prevention of type 2 diabetes (2).

1. Dryden, J. (2011, January 28). Researchers discover root cause of blood vessel damage in diabetes. Retrieved from https://source.wustl.edu/2011/01/researchers-discover-root-cause-of-blood-vessel-damage-in-diabetes/

2. Saini, V. (2010). Molecular mechanisms of insulin resistance in type 2 diabetes mellitus. World J Diabetes,1(3), 68-75. doi:10.4239/wjd.v1.i3.68

How can complex interactions of chronic diseases be simplified?

When considering the number of different chronic diseases, and their different combinations, it becomes evident that most are interrelated. The individual associations contribute to an overall association controlled by the disease mechanisms involved. Both the individual associations between chronic disease and the overall associations are important to help us understand disease prevention, pathology, and treatment. The disease interactions become very complex. Fortunately, there appears to be one main root cause of the major chronic diseases (unhealthy lifestyle) and therefore one overall prevention and treatment approach: healthy lifestyle. This converts a complex social and medical issue into a solvable problem (1).

> There appears to be one main root cause of the major chronic diseases (unhealthy lifestyle) and therefore one overall prevention and treatment approach: healthy lifestyle.

1. Schierer, T. (2016, September 3). Chronic effects of diabetes and its interaction with other chronic diseases [Web log post]. Retrieved from http://www.jettphc.com/chronic-effects-of-diabetes-and-its-interaction-with-other-chronic-diseases/

7

DIABETES RISK FACTORS AND REVERSIBILITY

Diabetes Risk Factors

DIABETES RISK FACTORS include physical, genetic, social, and environmental. They are mostly easy to assess. Even the genetic components are becoming easier to assess since the cost of DNA sequencing is so low. Genetic information is typically not needed to effectively treat an individual. As mentioned in the section on screening, quick assessments of weight and blood sugar are all that is needed to get started. Weight alone is enough information since the impact of obesity is known and is a metabolic disease itself.

Excess Weight: "Some experts believe obesity, especially excess fat around the waist, is a primary cause of insulin resistance. Scientists used to think that fat tissue functioned solely as energy storage. However, studies have shown that belly fat produces hormones and other substances that can cause serious health problems such as insulin resistance, high blood

pressure, imbalanced cholesterol, and cardiovascular disease"
(CVD) (1).

Belly fat: Belly fat is considered an active organ by doctors
in functional medicine. This is because it is involved in the
release of unwanted hormones, hunger signals from the brain,
and inflammatory signals (2). These signals initiate hunger
responses, slow metabolism, and promote fat storage, all of
which perpetuates the difficulty in losing belly fat. Belly fat
"plays a part in developing chronic, or long-lasting, inflammation in the body. Chronic inflammation can damage the
body over time, without any signs or symptoms. Scientists have
found that complex interactions in fat tissue draw immune cells
to the area and trigger low-level chronic inflammation. This
inflammation can contribute to the development of insulin
resistance, type 2 diabetes, and cardiovascular disease. Studies
show that losing the weight can reduce insulin resistance and
prevent or delay type 2 diabetes" (1).

Physical Inactivity: "Many studies have shown that physical
inactivity is associated with insulin resistance, often leading to
type 2 diabetes. In the body, more glucose is used by muscle
than other tissues. Normally, active muscles burn their stored
glucose for energy and refill their reserves with glucose taken
from the bloodstream, keeping blood glucose levels in balance.

"Studies show that after exercising, muscles become more sensitive to insulin, reversing insulin resistance and lowering blood
glucose levels. Exercise also helps muscles absorb more glucose
without the need for insulin. The more muscle a body has, the
more glucose it can burn to control blood glucose levels" (1).

1.   National Institute of Diabetes and Digestive and Kidney
Diseases. (n.d.). Prediabetes & insulin resistance.
National Institute of Diabetes and Digestive and Kidney

Diseases. Retrieved from https://www.niddk.nih.gov/health-information/diabetes/overview/what-is-diabetes/prediabetes-insulin-resistance

2. Hyman, M. (n.d.). 10 day detox diet starter kit. Retrieved from http://www.10daydetoxcookbook.com/?a_aid=54ef3e65242a0&a_bid=944fd4dd&chan=code4

Question: What are your non-genetic risk factors?

T2D Genetics

Behavioral level: Genetics make some patients more susceptible to the consequences of unhealthy diets. Genes associated with early onset of type 2 diabetes have been discovered that predisposed some people to type 2 diabetes onset before the age of 40. A study on Caucasians in France found a novel susceptibility locus for type 2 diabetes on chromosome 3q27-qter and confirmed the previously reported diabetes-susceptibility locus on chromosome 1q21-q24 (1).

Another group discovered mutations in either the HNF-1α or the HNF-4α genes which are present among the individuals who develop early-onset diabetes. A defect in insulin secretion is the hallmark in Mexican diabetic patients diagnosed between 20 and 40 years of age (2).

Genetically, some can tolerate a level of glucose in their diet and sedentary behavior that will harm others. Only about 30% of overweight people develop T2D.

MODY genetic study: The most common monogenic form of T2D is maturity-onset diabetes of the young (MODY). A study including researchers from Harvard and MIT's Broad Institute demonstrated that MODY genes "contribute little to the common form of the disease" (3).

1. Vionnet, N., et al. (2000). Genomewide search for type 2 diabetes–susceptibility genes in French whites: Evidence for a novel susceptibility locus for early-onset diabetes on chromosome 3q27-qter and independent replication of a type 2–diabetes locus on chromosome 1q21–q24. The American Journal of Human Genetics, 67(6), 1470-1480. doi:10.1086/316887

2. Aguilar-Salinas, C. A., et al. (2001). Early-onset type 2 diabetes: Metabolic and genetic characterization in the Mexican population. The Journal of Clinical Endocrinology & Metabolism, 86(1), 220-226. doi:10.1210/jcem. 86.1.7134

3. Winckler, W., et al. (2007). Evaluation of common variants in the six known maturity-onset diabetes of the young (MODY) genes for association with type 2 diabetes. Diabetes, 56(3), 685-693. https://doi.org/10.2337/ db06-0202

Question: What are your genetic risk factors?

Lifestyle has a much greater impact than genetics

If the genetic component had the biggest impact, the normal weight population would get T2D at a rate that corresponded to genetics rather than weight. In this scenario, genetics would mostly account for the 50% rate of prediabetes and diabetes. More genes that contribute to T2D will be found, but what is the relevance if T2D is mostly addressed through lifestyle and is 100% preventable? The ease of reversing prediabetes and early stage T2D clarifies that lifestyle has a much greater impact than genetics. T2D reversal rate increases dramatically with the level of weight loss. According to a study by Steven et al., reversal of diabetes was observed in (1):

> 80% of those who lost more than 20 kg reversed diabetes.

- 80% of those with > 20 kg weight loss
- 63% of those with 10–20 kg weight loss
- 53% of those with < 10 kg weight loss

Stanford Research Study: Relationship of sugar and high fructose corn syrup to diabetes prevalence

The Relationship of Sugar to Population-Level Diabetes Prevalence: An Econometric Analysis of Repeated Cross-Sectional Data (2)

This Stanford study is remarkable in terms of the high number of significant and specific findings with respect to the impact of sugar on diabetes prevalence. It used data on diabetes and nutritional components of food from 175 countries. Sugar was singled out as capable of independently increasing diabetes prevalence after testing for potential selection biases and controlling for other food types (including fibers, meats, fruits, oils, cereals), total calories, overweight and obesity, period-effects, and several socioeconomic variables such as aging, urbanization, and income.

Sugar "correlated significantly with diabetes prevalence in a dose-dependent manner, while declines in sugar exposure correlated with significant subsequent declines in diabetes rates.

"No other food types yielded significant individual associations with diabetes prevalence after controlling for obesity and other confounders." "The impact of sugar on diabetes was independent of sedentary behavior and alcohol use, and the effect was modified but not confounded by obesity or overweight." Sugar "correlated significantly with diabetes prevalence in a dose-dependent manner, while declines in sugar exposure correlated with significant subsequent declines in diabetes rates. This finding was independent of other socio-economic, dietary and obesity prevalence changes." Differences in sugar availability "statistically explain variations in diabetes prevalence rates." Diabetes rates are rising dramatically irrespective of obesity in many developing countries: Philippines, Romania, France, Bangladesh, and Georgia.

Stanford Study Findings (2)
One can of soda/day increased diabetes prevalence 1%
Other food types did not associate with increased diabetes prevalence
Non-food factors such as sedentary behavior did not affect singular ability of sugar to increase diabetes prevalence
As sugar consumption increases, so does diabetes onset
Differences in sugar availability "statistically explain variations in diabetes prevalence rates"
The sugar effect has the same trend with different ethnic compositions, indicating that this trend does not depend on culture or race

1. Steven, S., Lim, E. L., & Taylor, R. (2013). Population response to information on reversibility of type 2 diabetes. Diabetic Medicine, 30(4), e135-e138. doi:10.1111/dme.12116

2. Basu, S., Yoffe, P., Hills, N., & Lustig, R. H. (2013). The relationship of sugar to population-level diabetes prevalence: An econometric analysis of repeated cross-sectional data. PLoS One, 8(2), e57873.

Question: How much sugar do you consume each day? Have you measured it?

Psychological factors involved in T2D

> People do not feel physical symptoms in early stages. Therefore, they do not usually seek medical assistance or think a problem exists.

Awareness and food dependency issues important factors in diabetes onset. Awareness is particularly important because pre-diabetes in early-stage T2D are asymptomatic. People do not feel physical symptoms in early stages. Therefore, they do not usually seek medical assistance or think a problem exists. (1) This can occur with or without a doctor's advice. A significant proportion of the population do not see their doctor on a regular basis. Many of those who see their doctor do not respond to the doctor's advice. To complicate the situation even further, significant numbers of doctors and dietitians are still recommending high-carb, low-fat foods, albeit a healthier version than the food pyramids of the 1990s (2).

Lack of awareness of T2D
Pre-diabetics: 90% of pre-diabetics don't know they have pre-diabetes (1)
Diabetes: About 33% of those with diabetes don't know they have it (3)

1. Diabetes in the U.S., a Snapshot. (n.d.). Retrieved May, 2017, from http://www.cdc.gov/media/DPK/2014/ images/diabetes-report/Infographic1-web.pdf
2. Haspel, T. (2015). Is it really worth not eating bread, pasta and other carbs? Retrieved from https://

www.washingtonpost.com/national/health-science/
is-it-really-worth-not-eating-bread-pasta-and-other-
carbs/2015/02/06/cd6d1c38-89e2-11e4-a085-
34e9b9f09a58_story.html?utm_term=.b2dfd4d28a4c

3. One-Third of Adults with Diabetes Still Don't Know
    They Have It. (2006). Retrieved from http://www.nih.
    gov/news/pr/may2006/niddk-26.htm

Question: What can you do to increase your level of awareness?

What facilitates T2D lack of awareness?

Food addiction: Food addiction occurs when foods rich in fat and sugar overwhelm the brain's reward system and inhibit the brain's ability to instruct an individual to stop eating. According to Paul Kenny, Associate Professor at the Scripps Research Institute, obesity shares the following characteristics in common with alcohol and drug addiction (1):

- Obese people overeat for short-term pleasure, attempt to abstain, and then relapse—the same general pattern observed for drug addiction.

- Obese people develop tolerance (to appetite suppressing hormones).

- The more obese people eat, the more they want. Obese individuals must increase food consumption to overcome reduced activation of the brain's reward networks.

- Weight loss can trigger negative mood and depression in obese people—similar to withdrawal in addicts during abstinence.

- Drugs of abuse stimulate the brain's reward systems the way food does.

- It appears that obesity is caused by an overpowering motivation to satisfy the brain's reward centers.

- Endorphin blockers that help reduce heroin, cocaine, and alcohol use in human addicts also reduce food consumption in test subjects.

- Obese rats treated with endorphin blockers display behavior closely related to withdrawal.

- Obese individuals, alcoholics, and cocaine addicts all have low levels of a dopamine D2 receptor.

1. Kenny, P. J. (2013). The food addiction. Scientific American, 309, 44-49. doi:10.1038/scientificamerican0913-44

Question: Which items in the list above did you relate to?

Social factors involved in T2D

Overeating is one of the most common personal recovery issues. For a number of reasons, handling obesity is more complex than instructing individuals to eat less and exercise more. It is difficult for obese people to get the treatment and environment they need to become healthy. It is socially acceptable to over-consume the wrong types of food. Resisting overconsumption is very difficult because the wrong kind of food is continually offered by friends, associates, and the marketplace. Social acceptability facilitates denial of food addiction. We cannot treat what we are not aware of.

<table>
<tr><td align="center">Treatability
An unknown condition is not treatable</td></tr>
</table>

Question: How can you help your family and friends encourage your new health behaviors?

Environmental factors involved in T2D

Predominant foods and food choice The existence of saturation exposure to the wrong foods (high sugar, high in processed fat, high salt, high carb) creates an environment where change for the overeater is very difficult to achieve. In addition to being offered the wrong foods by friends and colleagues, the constant availability of the unhealthy foods and drinks at convenience stores, restaurants, and grocery stores decreases the chances of change. The typical American diet contains about 50% carbohydrates, including high levels of simple carbohydrates. Every time an overeater encounters a tempting food, they have to make a choice. As the number of encounters with the wrong types of food increases, so does the likelihood that unhealthy foods will be consumed. Most people become overweight as they gain a few pounds every year.

Why do diabetics lose limbs and eyesight?

As diabetes progresses to late stages, it can lead to blindness, amputation, and heart disease.

Diabetes impacts normal functionality at a high level and in several different areas:

- Eyes: Ability to read, drive, take pictures, and participate in sports that require vision.

- Feet: Mobility at work and at home and ability to walk, run, and play sports.

- Heart: Vital body organ - Diabetes is a top risk factor for heart disease.

- Kidneys: Vital body organ - Diabetes is a leading cause of kidney disease. The kidneys extract waste from blood, balance body fluids, and form urine. These functions can be impaired by kidney disease.

- Blood vessel problems are a common complication of diabetes. There are several different manifestations of blood vessel damage, including amputations, heart attack, stroke, and vision loss. Two of these end stages will be discussed as examples: vision loss and amputation.

How does diabetes lead to vision loss?

> Diabetes affects virtually all structures of the eye.

Diabetes affects virtually all structures of the eye. Many people experience blurred vision in the early stages of diabetes. This blurred vision is caused by fluid seeping into the lens of the eye and causing the lens to swell. Swelling changes its shape and alters its ability to focus properly. Once blood glucose is under control, the lens resumes its normal shape and vision improves. The fluid seepage is treatable and not permanent.

Blurred vision also can occur during insulin treatment or with fluctuating blood glucose levels. Again, fluids in the body are shifting, and fluid may enter or leave the lens. This condition is not permanent and usually lasts a few days or weeks. As blood glucose returns to normal, vision should improve. As a result, it is usually recommended that you wait until your blood glucose level and your vision stabilizes before getting or changing an eyeglass prescription.

Vision loss in diabetics is most often a result of diabetic retinopathy. Diabetic retinopathy involves bleeding or leakage of the blood vessels in the retina—the light-sensitive lining at the back of the eye. This leakage causes the retinal tissue to swell and distorts vision. According to the American Optometric Association, "diabetic retinopathy is the most common cause of vision loss among people with diabetes and a leading cause of blindness among working-age adults" (1).

Symptoms of diabetic retinopathy include:

- Seeing spots or floaters
- Blurred vision
- Having a dark or empty spot in the center of your vision
- Difficulty seeing well at night

The progression of diabetic retinopathy is not inevitable. Diabetics who can better control their blood sugar levels will slow the onset of diabetic retinopathy. Early stages of diabetic retinopathy are visually asymptomatic but can be detected by an optometrist. The American Optometric Association recommends that everyone with diabetes have a comprehensive dilated eye examination once a year. "Early detection and treatment can limit the potential for significant vision loss from diabetic retinopathy" (1).

If you are diabetic, you can help prevent or slow the development of diabetic retinopathy by (1):

- Taking prescribed medication
- Eating a healthy diet
- Exercising regularly
- Controlling high blood pressure

- Avoiding alcohol and smoking

1. American Optometric Association. (n.d.). Diabetic retinopathy. Retrieved from http://www.aoa.org/patients-and-public/eye-and-vision-problems/glossary-of-eye-and-vision-conditions/diabetic-retinopathy?sso=y

What are the symptoms of eye disease?

Diabetes has a strong impact on three of the four most common eye diseases in senior citizens (1,2). Diabetics are more prone to glaucoma, cataracts and other eye conditions. The following symptoms of eye disease need immediate attention (2):

- Sudden loss of vision.
- Severe eye pain.
- The sensation that a curtain is coming down over your eyes.
- Black or red floating spots in your vision.
- Distortion or waviness of straight lines.

Your eyes can become damaged without your awareness, because the damage can occur in areas that do not affect vision and you often feel no pain. According to the Joslin Center at Harvard, only careful eye examinations at regular intervals will detect the damage. Recommendations for eye exams are as follows (2):

- If you have type 1 diabetes, have your eyes examined by an eye doctor at least once a year.
- If you have type 2 diabetes, have your eyes examined when your diabetes is diagnosed and at least once a year afterward.

1. Sollitto, M. (n.d.). The 4 most common age-related eye diseases. AgingCare.com. Retrieved from https://www.agingcare.com/articles/the-4-most-common-age-related-eye-diseases-145190.htm

2. Joslin Diabetes Center. (n.d.). Symptoms of eye disease. Retrieved from http://www.joslin.org/info/Symptoms_of_Eye_Disease.html

Are diabetics more prone to glaucoma and cataracts?

Diabetics are more prone to getting glaucoma than non-diabetics. Glaucoma is caused by too much pressure in the eye. This pressure damages the optic nerve. Everyone past age 40 is at risk for glaucoma. "However, a person with diabetes may be nearly twice as likely to get glaucoma as other adults" (1). An ophthalmologist or optometrist can diagnose glaucoma by measuring eye pressure. If detected, glaucoma can be treated with prescription eye drops that cause proper fluid exchange or with laser treatments or other surgery if necessary. Glaucoma can progress and cause irreversible eye damage if it is not treated.

People with diabetes are also more likely to develop cataracts at a younger age. Cataracts are a condition in which the lens of the eye becomes clouded, blocking the transmission of light. This problem usually comes with advanced age. Poor blood sugar control can speed up the process of developing cataracts. Cataracts are treatable with surgery.

1. Joslin Diabetes Center. (n.d.). Diseases of the eye. Retrieved from http://www.joslin.org/info/Diseases_of_the_Eye.html

Does diabetes lead to amputations?

According to WebMD, "blood vessel and nerve damage linked with diabetes can lead to serious infections that are extremely hard to treat." Nerve damage makes it difficult to feel the feet and other areas that experience nerve damage. Feet are prone to injury when you lose the ability to feel them. As a result, feet are easily injured without knowing it. Serious infections can develop from minor injuries such as a small cut. These infections are capable of spreading up into the leg. If the infection is severe enough, the foot, and/or part of the leg must be amputated (1). Proper diabetes management and foot care can help prevent foot ulcers resulting in infection. Better diabetes care is likely the driver of a 50% decrease in the rates of lower limb amputations in the past 20 years (2).

One in four people with diabetes develops foot problems. The extreme cases require amputation. The amputation rate at the Joslin-Beth Israel Deaconess Foot Center has improved threefold since 1984: from 30% in 1984 to 8% currently. About 40% of people with diabetes develop neuropathy (nerve damage) (3). Once nerve death occurs, it is irreversible. However, prevention of further nerve damage is possible. For those with painful neuropathy, improved diabetes control and some medications can relieve the discomfort. Neuropathy is usually seen in people who have had diabetes more than 10 or 15 years. Those who haven't had good blood glucose control are particularly vulnerable. In addition to neuropathy, some diabetics develop vascular (blood vessel) disease. Without adequate blood flow, they may lose the ability to heal cuts or wounds. The injury problem is compounded because the ability to heal the wound is inhibited by poor circulation. For example, a minor callus can become infected, leading to an ulcer (an open wound) that, in turn, can lead to a more widespread infection and loss of part or all of the foot.

Initial treatment of foot ulcers always includes getting patients off their feet to relieve the foot's pressure points. Ulcers are often on the pressure points—the ball or heel of the foot. If necessary, the ulcer is debrided—that is, infected tissue is removed. In difficult cases when healing isn't occurring, "living skin equivalents" can be used to cover the wound. Topical growth factors can be applied to jumpstart healing of the tissue. The cause is identified in order to reduce the likelihood of recurrence. Problem shoes can be modified or replaced. If a foot deformity like a bunion or hammertoe is present, the patient may need corrective surgery. If the patient has vascular disease, surgeons can restore blocked circulation through bypass surgery. Angioplasty and stenting procedures are less invasive and may be used to clear the blockage in blood vessels. The only cases at the Joslin foot center that end in amputation occur when bypasses can't be performed for some reason, or when an infection has already caused too much bone and tissue loss.

Risk of vascular complications can be reduced through control of diet, blood pressure and lipid levels, and by not smoking cigarettes. People with diabetes should learn how to inspect their feet carefully and frequently, or have a helper do it for them. According to Dr. John Giurini, "I tell my patients that if they have lost the sensation of pain, they have to use another sense—their sight— to take its place. I advise them to look for any blisters, sores, swelling or cracks between the toes, and if they have pressure points, to wear padded socks or put inserts in their shoes. Everyone with diabetes should see a podiatrist at least once a year." Joslin does a series of examinations to check the status of circulation in the legs, nerve function and a simple two-minute "monofilament test" to assess if there is any protective sensation left in the foot. These diagnostics determine if someone is at risk for ulceration. Foot ulcers are common but quite preventable. The bottom line: if you take care of your feet, amputations are preventable.

1. WebMD. (n.d.). Diabetes: Amputation for foot problems – topic overview. Retrieved from http://www.webmd.com/diabetes/tc/amputation-for-diabetic-foot-problems-topic-overview

2. Mayo Clinic Staff. (2014). Amputation and diabetes: How to protect your feet: Good diabetes management and regular foot care help prevent severe foot sores that are difficult to treat and may require amputation. Mayo Clinic. Retrieved from http://www.mayoclinic.org/diseases-conditions/diabetes/in-depth/amputation-and-diabetes/art-20048262

3. Giurini, J. (n.d.). Foot care: Tips for keeping you on your toes. Retrieved from http://www.joslin.org/docs/foot_care_time_insert_11-2004.pdf

T2D reversibility

Treatment is the path most often taken instead of prevention. Treatment in the absence of behavior change allows us to keep the behaviors that lead to type 2 diabetes. In the end, treatment is much, much harder. The effects of obesity generate prolonged pain in many different areas. Taken together over time, the sum of these effects is much greater than the acute, short-term pain of healthy choices. The NIH has an excellent summary of the biological basis of the impact of healthy lifestyle changes on T2D (1).

What is the impact of healthy lifestyle change on physical health (1,2)?

Lifestyle change	Impact
Weight Loss	Improved beta cell function
Weight Loss	Decreases the need for treatment
Weight Loss and Exercise	Prevent insulin resistance

1. National Institute of Diabetes and Digestive and Kidney Diseases. (n.d.). Prediabetes & insulin resistance. National Institute of Diabetes and Digestive and Kidney Diseases. Retrieved from https://www.niddk.nih.gov/health-information/diabetes/overview/what-is-diabetes/prediabetes-insulin-resistance

2. Fonseca, V.A. (2009). Defining and characterizing the progression of type 2 diabetes. Diabetes Care, 32(Suppl 2), S151-S156. doi:10.2337/dc09-S301

How reversible is T2D?

Case Studies

How often can short-duration T2D patients reverse T2D (1)? Up to 80% of study subjects losing over 44 pounds achieved T2D reversal. This includes people who had T2D for varying lengths of time. Overall, up to 73% of study subjects who lost weight through lifestyle changes achieved a reversal of T2D.

How often can people who have T2D for several years reverse it (1)? 43% of those with T2D for over 8 years achieved reversal. This reflects the progressive nature of T2D. It also provides hope for those with T2D. Almost half of those who have had T2D for an extended period can still achieve reversal.

What is the longest T2D duration that still allows reversal (2)? Studies have shown that T2D reversal can be achieved after a T2D duration of at least 18 years. The demonstration that new beta cells can be developed from adult exocrine pancreatic ducts suggests that recovery of insulin secretion in long-duration diabetes is at least possible. A decline in beta cell function over time is to be expected, but it is not inevitable and is highly variable between individuals. Because the date of onset is "notoriously" inaccurate and usually late, the actual timespan within which reversal is achieved usually increases.

Case Study Summary

Weight Loss	Reversal Rate	Duration of T2D	Reversal Rate
>20 kg/44 lb	80%	< 4 years	73%
10–20 kg/ 22–44 lb	63%	4–8 years	56%
< 10 kg/ 22 lb	53%	> 8 years	43%

This case study clearly indicates that the chances of T2D reversal increase dramatically with the amount of weight lost. As mentioned previously, those with extreme obesity are recommended to lose at least 100 lb (3).

Increased duration of T2D requires greater degrees of weight loss (2). According to a study in the UK, in order to achieve reversal of T2D in patients who have had T2D for an extended period, "a greater degree of weight loss is required than for short-duration diabetes." Long duration patients who lost less than 25 kg (55 lbs) did significantly worse than short duration patients who were in the same weight loss category.

There was a notable lack of reversal in patients achieving < 25kg weight loss.

How does T2D reversal take place?	
Behavioral	Biological
Removal of belly fat	Normalization of beta cell function
Calorie restriction	Normalization of hepatic insulin sensitivity

According to a UK study in Diabetic Medicine, the data provide further evidence that removal of belly fat allows the return of normal metabolic function" (2). Some studies assert that calorie restriction alone can reverse Type 2 diabetes. Normalization of both beta cell function and hepatic insulin sensitivity in type 2 diabetes was achieved by dietary energy restriction alone. Insulin sensitivity increases in the first 7 days of lowering calorie intake to recommended levels. During this period, liver triglyceride content falls, and hepatic insulin sensitivity increases. The recovery in beta-cell function is likely to relate to removal of the burden of the toxic metabolites of saturated fatty acids.

Characteristics of those not achieving reversal in spite of significant weight loss (2)
Older
Longer diabetes duration
Higher preoperative BMI and preoperative HbA1c levels
More likely to be on insulin or glucagon-like peptide-1 agonist therapies than those who did achieve a postoperative HbA1c of < 43 mmol/mol (6.1%)

These individuals did not achieve a non-diabetic HbA1c of < 6.1% (43 mmol/mol) despite weight loss of > 25kg. The main lessons here are to test early, test regularly, and reverse T2D as soon as possible.

1. Steven, S., Lim, E. L., & Taylor, R. (2013). Population response to information on reversibility of type 2 diabetes. Diabetic Medicine, 30(4), e135-e138. doi:10.1111/dme.12116

2. Steven, S., Carey, P. E., Small, P. K., & Taylor, R. (2014). Reversal of type 2 diabetes after bariatric surgery is determined by the degree of achieved weight loss in both short- and long-duration diabetes. Diabetic Medicing, 32(1): 47-53. doi:10.1111/dme.12567

3. WebMD. (2015). Tips to lose 100 pounds or more. Retrieved from http://www.webmd.com/diet/features/10-tips-losing-100-pounds-or-more

8
DIABETES REVERSAL TESTING

90% of pre-diabetics don't know

THE EPIDEMIC OF type 2 diabetes had taken hold in the United States by the late 1990s. The epidemic has spread throughout the world. Lack of awareness has impacted this issue in very significant ways. The lack of awareness in the scientific community regarding differentiation of caloric quality and the value of healthy fats led to erroneous diet recommendations that greatly augmented the type 2 epidemic. Scientists and citizens all believed that all fat was bad and that all calories were created equal.

The need for individuals to regularly test their blood sugar is another area that lacked awareness. Most prediabetics live a normal life in spite of their pre-diabetic condition. It turns out that over 90% of prediabetics are unaware or unconcerned that their blood sugar reading indicates that they have pre-diabetes (1). Blood sugar testing is an essential component to reversing the epidemic of type 2 diabetes.

If you have friends, coworkers, and family who exhibit some of the risk factors for diabetes, ask them if they had their blood sugar tested. Inexpensive blood sugar meters are available at drugstores for as little as $10. The combination of faulty nutritional research, faulty nutritional recommendations and lack of testing has been a potent driving force for the diabetes epidemic. The reverse approach should be able to counter or slow the progress of the epidemic. This reversal has begun.

1. American Diabetes Association. (n.d.). Type 2. http://www.diabetes.org/diabetes-basics/type-2/?loc=util-header_type2

The importance of blood sugar testing

> The lack of awareness of blood glucose levels is a serious condition in America where 50% are pre-diabetic or diabetic.

The lack of awareness of blood glucose levels is a serious condition in America where 50% are pre-diabetic or diabetic (1). This lack of awareness facilitates the development of a progressive disease state in which hidden damage to the body is occurring slowly over time. It is estimated that damage to the body occurs over 10 years before diagnosis of diabetes.

Awareness of one's diabetic risk is useful for prevention and recovery from the disease. The sooner people begin to reverse type 2 diabetes, the greater their chances of recovery. In one study, those who began to address diabetes within 4 years of diagnosis had greater than a 70% chance of reversal whereas those waiting longer than 8 years had less than a 45% chance of reversal (3).

The high rates of pre-diabetes and diabetes make blood sugar testing a very high priority for Americans. Inexpensive test kits are available at drugstores, and free blood sugar testing is often done at health fairs and places of employment. Because the symptoms of pre-diabetes often go unnoticed, most people do not get tested. You can greatly facilitate your own long-term health by getting your blood sugar tested on a regular basis and by consulting wellness professionals about the quality of your diet.

Rationale for blood sugar testing

- 50% of Americans are pre-diabetic or diabetic (1)

- 90% of pre-diabetics are unaware of their potential to develop diabetes (2)

- 33% of Americans are predicted to develop diagnosed type 2 diabetes by 2050 (4)

- Type 2 diabetes reversal can help alleviate other diet driven diseases

- The sooner a pre-diabetic or diabetic begins the reversal process, the greater the chances of success (3)

Blood sugar testing is needed on a wide scale. It is unlikely that our communities and healthcare systems will be able to support the estimated future levels of chronic disease. What are the major factors involved? The diabetes epidemic is burdensome to the healthcare system by itself. In addition to diabetes, there are several diabetes-related chronic diseases that add to the burden on our communities and healthcare facilities, including obesity, heart disease, kidney disease, cancer, autoimmune disease, and Alzheimer's.

Problems can lead to solutions by reversing the direction of the problem trend. Diabetes exacerbates a series of chronic diseases. Reversing diabetes is a major factor in reversing this series of chronic disease epidemics throughout the world (5,6).

The advantages of targeting diabetes include:

- The path to recovery is known

- Diabetes can serve as a focal point for reversal of a series of diet-based chronic disease

1. Crawford, C. (2015). JAMA study finds half of U.S. adults have diabetes or prediabetes. American Academy of Family Physicians. Retrieved from http://www.aafp.org/news/health-of-the-public/20150918jamadiabetes.html

2. Centers for Disease Control and Prevention. (n.d.). Diabetes. Retrieved October 3, 2017, from https://www.cdc.gov/chronicdisease/resources/publications/aag/diabetes.htm

3. Steven, S., Lim, E. L., & Taylor, R. (2013). Population response to information on reversibility of type 2 diabetes. Diabetic Medicine, 30(4), e135-e138. doi:10.1111/dme.12116

4. Boyle, J. P. et al. (2010). Projection of the year 2050 burden of diabetes in the US adult population: dynamic modeling of incidence, mortality, and prediabetes prevalence. Popul Health Metr.,8(29), 1-12. doi:10.1186/1478-7954-8-29

5. Hyman, M. (2012). The blood sugar solution: The ultrahealthy program for losing weight, preventing disease, and feeling great now!. New York, NY: Little, Brown and Company.

6. Hyman, M. (2016). Eat fat, get thin: Why the fat we eat is the key to sustained weight loss and vibrant health. New York, NY: Little, Brown and Company.

Prediabetes can be detected with one of the following blood tests:

- HbA1C test

- Fasting plasma glucose (FPG) test

- Oral glucose tolerance test (OGTT)

The A1C test accurately reflects beta cell failure over time (1). It accurately reflects the decreased ability of the pancreas to function. It is the most accurate blood sugar test (1,2). The A1C test is the primary test used for diabetes management and diabetes research. HbA1c is not as sensitive as the other tests. In some individuals, it may miss prediabetes that the other glucose tests may catch. Some health care providers can quickly measure A1C in their office with a point-of-care test.

> The A1C test is the primary test used for diabetes management and diabetes research.

This test is not considered reliable for diagnosis. For diagnosis of prediabetes, the A1C test should be analyzed in a laboratory using a method that is certified by the NGSP, a standardization agency (3).

- A1C range for prediabetes: An A1C of 5.7 to 6.4 percent indicates prediabetes.

1. Diabetes. (n.d.). Retrieved July 14, 2017, from https://www.niddk.nih.gov/health-information/diabetes#resistance

2. The A1C Test & Diabetes. (n.d.). Retrieved July 14, 2017, from http://diabetes.niddk.nih.gov/dm/pubs/A1CTest

3. Harmonizing Hemoglobin A1C Testing. (2010).
    Retrieved July 14, 2017, from http://www.ngsp.org/

Question: What is your frequency of blood sugar testing?

Fasting plasma glucose test

This test measures blood glucose in people who have not eaten anything for at least 8 hours. This test is most reliable when done in the morning. Prediabetes discovered with this test is called impaired fasting glucose (IFG).

- IFG range for prediabetes: Fasting glucose levels of 100 to 125 mg/dL indicate prediabetes.

OGTT

This test measures blood glucose after people have fasted for at least 8 hours and 2 hours after they drink a sweet liquid provided by a health care provider or laboratory. Prediabetes found with this test is called IGT.

- A blood glucose level between 140 and 199 mg/dL indicates prediabetes.

Question: Which blood sugar tests have you done? What were the results?

Guidelines for an adult with diabetes:

- 70 to 130 mg/dL before breakfast
- less than 180 mg/dL 2 hours after meals
- A1C less than 7

- Joslin Diabetes Center. (n.d.). Goals for Blood Glucose Control. Retrieved November 5, 2017, from http://www.joslin.org/info/Goals-for-Blood-Glucose-Control.html

Exercise: How much does blood glucose vary among a large population?

According to WebMD, the following ranges provide perspective on prediabetic glucose levels and monitoring (1):

	Low ranges	Mid ranges	High ranges
	60–70	71–80	81–90
Your glucose			

"During the day, blood glucose levels tend to be at their lowest just before meals. For most people without diabetes, blood sugar levels before meals hover around 70 to 80 mg/dL. In some, 60 is normal; in others, 90. Again, anything less than 100 mg/dL while fasting is considered normal by today's standards.

What's a low sugar level? It varies widely, too. Many people's sugar levels won't ever fall below 60 mg/dL, even with prolonged fasting. When you diet or fast, the liver keeps sugar levels normal by turning fat and muscle into sugar. A few people's sugar levels may fall somewhat lower. Decreasing blood sugar too low is usually not a concern. According to WebMD, "it's difficult to drop sugar levels to an unsafe point" (1).

Testing is important because the transition from prediabetes to diabetes is rapid rather than gradual (2). It can occur within a 3-year time frame. 8.1% of subjects whose initial abnormal fasting glucose was 100–109 mg/dl and 24.3% of subjects whose initial normal fasting glucose was 110 –125 mg/dl developed diabetes over an average of 29.0 months.

1. WebMD. (n.d.). High blood sugar, diabetes, and your body. Retrieved from http://www.webmd.com/diabetes/how-sugar-affects-diabetes

2. Fonseca, V.A. (2009). Defining and characterizing the progression of type 2 diabetes. Diabetes Care, 32(Suppl 2), S151-S156. doi:10.2337/dc09-S301

Question: Have you seen examples of a rapid transition? What did you observe?

How can an accurate, long range average of blood glucose be obtained?

HbA1c is an accurate measure of blood glucose. The term HbA1c is in regard to glycated hemoglobin. Hemoglobin (Hb) is a protein within red blood cells (RBCs) that carries oxygen throughout your body. When Hb joins with glucose in the blood, it is 'glycated' (1).

Because red blood cells are being generated continuously, every blood sample represents an average of the starting points of the population of cells in the sample. There are millions of red blood cells in 2-3 drops of blood (2). These red blood cells all started at different times (about 2 million are generated per second). This multitude of cells represent essentially every possible starting point in the 8 to 12 weeks regeneration time. HbA1c is like taking a blood glucose reading multiple times per day during the 8 to 12 weeks and computing the average.

Conversely, direct measurement of blood glucose from a single time point after fasting 12 hours represents the results of what you ate within the last few days. It takes about 10 days to detox the blood from a poor diet. Fasting blood glucose has usefulness for determining the impact of diet on short-term blood glucose levels. It is a relatively poor measurement of overall long-term blood glucose levels.

1. Guide to HbA1c. (n.d.). Retrieved July 14, 2017, from http://www.diabetes.co.uk/what-is-hba1c.html

2. Whole Blood and Red Blood Cells. (n.d.). Retrieved July 14, 2017, from http://www.redcrossblood. org/learn-about-blood/blood-components/ whole-blood-and-red-blood-cells

How to determine the impact of your diet on blood glucose

When we eat, the digestive system breaks down the carbo-hydrates into various sugar molecules. Glucose is the body's principal source of energy. Glucose can only enter cells if insulin in the bloodstream triggers glucose entry. Without insulin, the cells would starve (1).

The impact of our diet on blood glucose can be determined by a handheld blood glucose meter. This type of test is the one we see when people take a measurement at a restaurant or a shopping center. The blood glucose meter measures the amount of glucose in the blood as determined by an enzymatic reaction with reagents on a test strip. The reaction generates electrons, resulting in an electric current proportional to the glucose in the sample. The meter then calculates a glucose concentration and displays it.

Food and drink containing high levels of simple carbohydrates do not need to be digested in order for blood glucose levels to rise. Free glucose is already present in these items, and it enters the blood directly from the digestive system (1). A glucose meter test is a very useful measurement for determining the immediate impact of any kind of food or drink on blood glucose.

1. Nordqvist, C. (2017). Blood sugar or blood glucose: What does it do?. Medical News Today. Retrieved from http://www.medicalnewstoday.com/articles/249413.php

How to accurately test blood sugar

In order to accurately assess blood sugar, several considerations must be made (1):

- Wash and dry hands to remove any residues from lotion or sugar in our food that may impact the result.

- Test blood from your finger: Blood from the non-finger parts of the arm doesn't reflect your current blood glucose level. "The blood circulation to the rest of the arm takes longer than it does to the fingertips." If your blood glucose changes rapidly, only a finger-prick will do.

- Don't squeeze the blood out of the finger: Squeezing and rubbing your finger after you've pricked it can affect the blood sample. "Sometimes you'll get a little more interstitial fluid [the substance just below the skin] than the capillary blood." Washing with warm water will increase blood flow to the fingers, making it easier to get blood without squeezing.

- Coded meters require a number or use a "key" or "chip" each time you open a new bottle of test strips. Anytime you think your meter is making mistakes, make sure your meter has the code from your current test strip bottle.

- Use control solution to verify the accuracy of the meter: If you get a reading that seems inaccurate—test how well the meter is working by using the meter's control solution. If you can't find your meter's brand of solution at the pharmacy, ask your pharmacist to order it. Make sure your control solution isn't expired.

- Use unexpired test strips: Discard outdated test strips since they may be unreliable.

- Ensure proper storage of test strips and meter: Improper storage of strips will yield poor results. Don't store your meter and strips where it's too hot, too cold, too humid, or too high in altitude (meters and strips should perform in pressurized airplanes).

1. Neithercott, T. (2012). 10 ways to master your blood glucose meter. Diabetes Forecast. Retrieved from http://www.diabetesforecast.org/2012/apr/10-ways-to-master-your-blood-glucose-meter.html

How to determine the level of insulin resistance in your body

Insulin resistance is one of the key factors in the development of type 2 diabetes. Thus, it is very important to measure the level of insulin. An insulin assay may be done when an individual has or is suspected of having insulin resistance, including people with type 2 diabetes, polycystic ovarian syndrome (PCOS), prediabetes or heart disease, or metabolic syndrome (1).

A 2-hour glucose tolerance test (GTT) can help determine the level of insulin resistance. First, a fasting glucose test is performed to establish a baseline. A GTT is done next, starting with the patient drinking a 75-gram glucose drink. A blood sample is drawn 2 hours after the glucose drink. This 'challenges' the person's body to process the glucose. "Normally, the blood glucose level rises after the drink and stimulates the pancreas to release insulin into the bloodstream and falls as insulin stimulates glucose uptake by cells." "When a person is unable to produce enough insulin, or if the body's cells are resistant to its effects (insulin resistance), less glucose is transported from the blood into cells, and the blood glucose level remains high" (2).

The level of insulin resistance is estimated from the blood glucose level (3):

- "A normal blood glucose level is lower than 140 mg/dL (7.8 mmol/L).

- A blood glucose level between 140 mg/dL and 199 mg/dL (7.8 and 11 mmol/L) is considered impaired glucose tolerance, or prediabetes. If you have prediabetes, you're at risk of eventually developing type 2 diabetes. You're also at risk of developing heart disease, even if you don't develop diabetes.

- A blood glucose level of 200 mg/dL (11.1 mmol/L) or higher may indicate diabetes."

1. Lab Tests Online. (2015). Insulin. Retrieved from https://labtestsonline.org/understanding/analytes/insulin/tab/test/

2. Lab Tests Online. (2017). Glucose tests. Retrieved from https://labtestsonline.org/understanding/analytes/glucose/tab/test/

3. Mayo Clinic Staff. (2015). Glucose tolerance test. Mayo Clinic. Retrieved form http://www.mayoclinic.org/tests-procedures/glucose-tolerance-test/basics/results/prc-20014814

Why is it useful to measure insulin levels?

Insulin testing has several other possible uses. Insulin testing may be used to help (1):

- Diagnose an insulinoma (insulin production from a tumor), verify tumor removal has been successful, and/or to monitor for recurrence.

- Diagnose the cause of hypoglycemia (low blood sugar) in an individual with signs and symptoms.

- Identify insulin resistance.

- "Monitor the amount of insulin produced by the beta cells in the pancreas (endogenous); in this case, a C-peptide test may also be done. Insulin and C-peptide are produced by the body at the same rate as part of the conversion of proinsulin to insulin in the pancreas. Both tests may be ordered when a health practitioner wants to evaluate how much insulin in the blood is made by the body and how much is from outside (exogenous) sources such as insulin injections. The test for insulin measures insulin from both sources while the C-peptide test reflects insulin produced by the pancreas."

- "Determine when a type 2 diabetic might need to start taking insulin to supplement oral medications."

- "Determine and monitor the success of an islet cell transplant intended to restore the ability to make insulin, by measuring the insulin-producing capacity of the transplant."

The wide variety of useful information from insulin levels illustrates the importance of test data. One test can yield many insightful results. Without adequate testing, our true health status remains unknown.

1. Lab Tests Online. (2015). Insulin. Retrieved from https://labtestsonline.org/understanding/analytes/insulin/tab/test/

What are the most important tests for health and wellness?

The timing of health testing, the combination of tests performed, and the combination of information provided to the patient are all critical. It is like a three-legged stool. If one of the legs is removed or inadequate, the stool topples. Many people continue eating foods high in simple carbohydrates and other unhealthy sources because their blood panel is supposedly good. Then, a decade or two later, a series of health problems arises. These problems reinforce each other and worsen overall health unless addressed. Addressing health problems requires a multifaceted approach to a multifaceted problem. If any of the critical tests are missing, health can be deteriorating, even though a standard blood panel may indicate that a person is healthy.

This raises the question of whether standard blood panels are complete or enough? Standard blood panels provide information on HDLs and triglycerides, two of the most important risk factors for heart disease. However, they do not include LDL particle size information, and the results can actually mislead people. My lab results are an example of this. I have struggled with keeping my LDLs in the healthy range, probably because of genetics. They have risen over 160 (high risk) at least 5 times and were in the healthy range only three times in one 10-year period. I have struggled with LDLs, no matter what my diet is. When my LDLs were near normal range at 137 mg/dL, the LDL particle size test showed that my small and medium size LDL particles were well into the high range. However, my triglyceride/HDL ratio and insulin levels are ideal, and my diet has helped maintain this ideal state. These test results indicate that I have very low insulin resistance. It remains to be seen whether my excellent triglyceride/HDL will overcome my long struggle with LDL levels. Some prominent wellness scientists such as Dr. Barry Sears do not believe that LDL levels are nearly as important as triglyceride/ HDL (1).

> Triglycerides, HDLs, HbA1C and AA/EPA ratio are the most important measures of physical wellness.

The following is a recommended list of tests that can help reverse diabetes and gauge your level of wellness:

HbA1C

- Why: Reliable overall measure of blood glucose (2)

2 Hour glucose tolerance test

- Why: Indicates the level of insulin resistance (8)

Triglycerides/HDL ratio

- Why: Triglyceride/HDL ratio indicates whether an individual has metabolic syndrome and insulin resistance (1). High HDL are associated with heart health (7)

Cortisol

- Why: Indicator of stress-induced inflammation. The combination of cortisol, insulin levels, and AA/EPA give you a clear indication of your level of inflammation. This triad is one of the best indicators of overall wellness (1)

AA/EPA ratio

- Why: Determines the level of inflammation (1)
- Less expensive alternative tests for inflammation: Homocysteine (4) and C-reactive protein

Blood pressure

- Why: Blood vessel damage and risk of heart failure or stroke increase with prolonged exposure to high blood pressure.

LDL particle size count

- Why: Small, dense LDL particles correlate with heart disease (5, 6)

Gut testing

- Why: Gut infection is an important factor in determining the cause of high LDL particles levels and sources of inflammation (6)

Only a few of the tests listed above are typically part of standard blood profiles. According to current health science data, all of the above test measurements should be included in a standard panel. Health insurance may not cover the cost of several of the tests listed. However, it is inexpensive compared to the cost of a heart attack, stroke, or bypass surgery.

Range of heart bypass surgery costs: $50,000–$250,000 (9)

Cost of lost wages = Your salary x years unable to work

- E.g. $50,000 X 1 year = $50,000
- E.g. $200,000 X 10 years = $2,000,000
- E.g. $75,000 X rest of life (permanent disability) = ?

Most people can address bad test results through diet, exercise, and stress management. If your wellness efforts are following recommendations consistently and you still get a bad number, you can experiment with diet, supplements, or wellness behaviors until you find something that works. If nothing seems to work, maintain the good results that you have through the behaviors that are working.

1. Sears, B. (2005). The anti-inflammation zone: Reversing the silent epidemic that's destroying our health (The zone). New York, NY: HarperCollins Publishers Inc.

2. National Institute of Diabetes and Digestive and Kidney Disease. (2014). Retrieved from https://www.niddk.nih.gov/health-information/diabetes/diagnosis-diabetes-prediabetes/a1c-test

3. Mercola, J. (2001). Insulin and its metabolic effects. Retrieved from http://articles.mercola.com/sites/articles/archive/2001/07/14/insulin-part-one.aspx

4. Oudi, M. E., et al. (2010). Homocysteine and markers of inflammation in acute coronary syndrome.

5. Kresser, C. (2013). The diet-heart myth: Why everyone should know their LDL particle number. Retrieved from https://chriskresser.com/the-diet-heart-myth-why-everyone-should-know-their-ldl-particle-number/

6. Kresser, C. (2013). What causes elevated LDL particle number?. Retrieved from https://chriskresser.com/what-causes-elevated-ldl-particle-number/

7. Mayo Clinic Staff. (2016). HDL cholesterol: How to boost your 'good' cholesterol. Mayo Clinic. Retrieved from http://www.mayoclinic.org/diseases-conditions/high-blood-cholesterol/in-depth/hdl-cholesterol/art-20046388

8. Hyman, M. (n.d.). The one test your doctor isn't doing that could save your life. Dr. Hyman. Retrieved from http://drhyman.com/blog/2014/08/18/one-test-doctor-isnt-save-life/

9. Healthcare Bluebook. (n.d.). Fair price information. Retrieved from https://www.healthcarebluebook.com/page_ProcedureDetails.aspx?id=49&dataset=md&g=Coronary+Bypass+Surgery

Early Diagnosis and risk testing

Prevention over treatment: Perhaps the most obvious reason to undergo testing is that early diagnosis can prevent serious problems. We have all heard this message for a variety of conditions. It is particularly true for T2D. Studies show that the earlier T2D is addressed, the greater the reversal rate. T2D is a progressive disease. The longer people have T2D, the more damage is done. Current medications like metformin help reduce the impact of T2D, but there is no cure. Metformin is still the "first-line oral therapy for T2D" after decades of study, beginning in the 1950s (1). This emphasizes the importance of prevention over treatment. Reliance on treatment for a preventable condition is never the best path personally, or nationally.

> Studies show that the earlier T2D is addressed, the greater the reversal rate.

1. Viollet, B., et al. (2012). Cellular and molecular mechanisms of metformin: An overview. Clinical Science, 122(6), 253-270.

Exercise: Online risk test

The American Diabetes Association has an online test based upon risk factors for type 2 diabetes.

- Take the following risk factor test to determine your overall risk for type 2 diabetes:
  - o ADA online risk test: http://www.diabetes.org/are-you-at-risk/diabetes-risk-test/

- What is your response to your risk level and the next step guidelines?

- Share your response with someone you are in community with that you respect and trust. You can call this person your sponsor or accountability partner. How does their perspective help you?

9
PROGRAMS THAT FACILITATE REVERSAL OF DIABETES

Institute for Functional Medicine

DR. MARK HYMAN'S functional medicine program tests patients for nutritional and wellness needs and designs a specific diet for them. The focus of Dr. Hyman's diabetes program is movement from centralized healthcare to self-care. The program is summarized in The Blood Sugar Solution (1). Hyman's 10-Day Detox is recommended for the initial phase of diabetes reversal and The Blood Sugar Solution program is recommended for the main phase of diabetes reversal and physical health recovery. They are particularly effective at handling the cravings that drive diabetes. The 10-day program is scientifically designed to remove the chemicals in our bodies that drive cravings for sugar, caffeine, and the wrong kinds of fats.

Summary of functional medicine program

- *Testing and patient surveys* are used to determine nutritional imbalances and to customize a patient-specific plan for preventative healthcare.

- *Food as a drug:* Patient-specific diets are considered the best drug to improve nutrition, regulate hormones, reduce inflammation, improve digestion, maximize detoxification, and enhance metabolism.

- *Belly fat:* The role of belly fat in disease is addressed through diet, mind relaxation, and exercise.

- *Holistic lifestyle change* includes relaxation and community components to lifestyle change.

The Blood Sugar Solution (1) focuses on "healthy carbs, healthy fats, healthy protein, healing spices, drinks and super-foods." The guideline for any meal is 50–75% plate volume of non-starchy vegetables, 25% plate volume of healthy animal or vegetable protein, 25% plate volume starchy carbs, low glycemic fruit or non-gluten grains, 25-50% of total calories for healthy fat, and water or herbal teas to drink.

Characteristics of the Blood Sugar Solution diet

- Highest food quality
- Fresh organic vegetables and other ingredients
- Healthy oils: olive oil and coconut oil
- Nuts and seeds
- Low gluten or gluten-free
- Low dairy or dairy-free
- PGX plant fiber to slow sugar uptake and reduce insulin spikes

- High choice variety and high flavor quality

- Highest nutrition standards

- Fresh vegetables, low carbs, and lean meats with little to no processed ingredients

- 90/10 rule: Health is maintained as long as you stick to the plan 90% of the time. A 100% rule is probably impractical for most people, given travels schedules and food prep time

1. Hyman, M. (2012). The blood sugar solution: The ultrahealthy program for losing weight, preventing disease, and feeling great now!. New York, NY: Little, Brown and Company.

Some personal testimonies from functional medicine programs and high healthy fat programs are listed below:

Craving control

"My husband said that he didn't think I was on a diet—he said diets are full of deprivation and since I wasn't feeling deprived I couldn't call it a diet anymore. It does feel good not to be driven by my stomach! I feel so different in such a good way." This patient lost 22 pounds and decreased her waist 5 inches. Program: Dr. David Ludwig's *Always Hungry* program

- Ludwig, D. (2016). Always hungry: Conquer cravings, retrain your fat cells, and lose weight permanently. New York, NY: Grand Central Publishing.

"Eat Fat Get Thin is an awesome program! I never imagined how big a difference I would see in a mirror in 3 weeks and how much better I feel. Yesterday I even passed up dessert easily without regret! Thank you for giving me the tools to make the changes I need in life for my help!" Program: Dr. Mark Hyman's *Eat Fat, Get Thin* program

- Hyman, M. (2016). Eat fat, get thin: Why the fat we eat is the key to sustained weight loss and vibrant health. New York, NY: Little, Brown and Company.

Elimination of medications

"I was taking 200 units of Lantus insulin daily and my hemoglobin A1c average blood sugar was still over the top. I came off insulin the third day on the program lost 35 pounds so far, and my last hemoglobin A1c was down to 6.9 from over 11." Program: Dr. Mark Hyman's *Eat Fat, Get Thin* program

Mental clarity

"Initially giving up sweets was hard. But the program was perfect for me because you just ate what you like, but in smarter ways. Then, when I would eat pizza, soda, or popcorn, I would feel really gross. The program help me obtain a much healthier and smarter relationship with the food. I feel more mentally clear and just happier. I would recommend this program to anyone." Program: Dr. David Ludwig's Always Hungry program

Daniel Plan

The Daniel Plan (1) has very similar characteristics to Dr. Hyman's diabesity program at the Institute for Functional Medicine. The Daniel plan has a stronger community component but does not include testing as part of the program.

What are the characteristics of the Daniel Plan diet?

- 50% non-starchy veggies
- 25% whole grains
- 25% lean proteins
- Low simple sugars
- Low gluten
- Low dairy
- High veggie
- Healthy oils/No trans fats

Exercise: For those who have not been in the habit of exercise, the Daniel Plan provides an exercise plan that you can customize to your needs and maintain. The exercise recommendations include:

- Starting slowly
- Cross training to prevent overuse of the same joints
- Exercise variety to reduce chances of burnout
- Increases in exercise frequency and intensity as you improve
- Body rest when needed

Exercise programs are designed for longevity and still meet fitness standards. There is high flexibility regarding exercise intensity level. Those capable of high-intensity workouts can push themselves as hard as they want. This approach allows those who struggle with exercise to choose a program they can stick with for long-term improvement and increase intensity as they are able. The community component improves consistency, longevity, and the desire to improve.

1. Warren, R., Amen, D., & Hyman, M. (2013). The Daniel plan: 40 days to a healthier life. Grand Rapids, MI: Zondervan.

The Diabetes Prevention Program

The Diabetes Prevention Program (DPP) was a major multicenter clinical research study aimed at discovering whether modest weight loss through dietary changes and increased physical activity or treatment with the oral diabetes drug metformin (Glucophage) could prevent or delay the onset of type 2 diabetes in study participants (1,2).

Key Characteristics of DPP study (3)

- Clearly defined weight loss and physical activity goals
- Individual case managers or "lifestyle coaches"
- Intensive, ongoing intervention
- Initial core curriculum to achieve standardization of the intervention
- Supervised exercise sessions offered at least two times per week throughout the trial
- A flexible maintenance program with supplemental group classes, motivational campaigns, and restart opportunities
- Individualization through a variety of strategies
- Materials and strategies that addressed the needs of an ethnically diverse population
- An extensive local and national network of training, feedback, and clinical support

DPP Outcomes

"The study found that prevention or delay of type 2 diabetes with lifestyle intervention or metformin in a high-risk population, as seen in the DPP study, can persist for at least 10 years. After an average of 10 years follow-up, intensive lifestyle changes aimed at modest weight loss reduced the rate of developing type 2 diabetes by 34%, delayed type 2 diabetes by about 4 years, and reduced cardiovascular risk factors, hemoglobin A1c, and fasting glucose when compared with placebo."

1. The National Institute of Diabetes and Digestive and Kidney Diseases.(n.d.). Diabetes Prevention Program. Retrieved July 14, 2017 from https://www.niddkrepository.org/studies/dpp/

2. Diabetes Prevention Program Outcomes Study (DPPOS). (2001). Retrieved July 14, 2017, from https://www.niddkrepository.org/studies/dppos/

3. The Diabetes Prevention Program Research Group. (2002). The diabetes prevention program (DPP). Diabetes Care, 25(12), 2165-2171.

Gastric bypass study: Reversing diabetes within weeks or months based on diet alone

Gastric bypass patients are known to reverse diabetes in days or weeks. In order to determine if this was due to changes brought about by the surgery or changes in diet, researchers conducted a diabetes reversal study based on diet alone (1,2).

Reversal of type 2 diabetes: normalization of beta cell function in association with decrease pancreas and liver triglycerides

Reversal diet characteristics:

- Protein shake
- Low glycemic load
- Plant-based, low-calorie diet
- No exercise in order to isolate the effect of diet

Reversal study characteristics:

- Purpose: Measure the effect of diet change on diabetes reversal
- Parameters measured: researchers measured hallmarks of diabetes
  - blood sugar and insulin responses
  - cholesterol levels
  - fat in the pancreas and liver
- Time points of Measurement
  - Before diet change
  - After diet change at 1, 4, and 8 weeks

Gastric bypass diabetes reversal study results were as follows:

> Patients reversed most features of diabetes within one week and all features by eight weeks.

- Patients reversed most features of diabetes within one week and all features by eight weeks.
- Diet reversal was much better than medications: Medications do not reverse diabetes; they treat diabetes. If your diabetes reversal progresses through

diet, work with your doctor to determine when you can stop medication.

- Pancreatic beta cells— insulin producing cells—reactivated.

- Fat deposits in the pancreas and liver dissipated.

- Blood sugars normalized in one week.

- Triglycerides dropped in half in one week and reduced 10-fold in eight weeks.

- Body cells became more insulin-sensitive.

- In 8 weeks, all evidence of diabetes was gone, and the test results of the diabetic patients looked very similar to normal control patients.

1. Hyman, M. (n.d.). New research finds diabetes can be reversed. Dr. Hyman. Retrieved from http://drhyman.com/blog/2011/08/04/ new-research-finds-diabetes-can-be-reversed/

2. Lim, E. L., Hollingsworth, K. G., Aribisala, B. S., Chen, M. J., Mathers, J. C., & Taylor, R. (2011). Reversal of type 2 diabetes: Normalisation of beta cell function in association with decreased pancreas and liver triacylglycerol. Diabetologia, 54, 2506-2514. doi:10.1007/ s00125-011-2204-7

NEJM study (1)

A Finnish study in the New England Journal of Medicine (NEJM) by Tuomilehto et al. is one of the most cited studies concerning prevention of T2D through lifestyle intervention. The overall conclusion by the researchers was that type 2 diabetes can be prevented by changes in the lifestyles of both women and men at high risk for the disease. The overall incidence of diabetes was reduced by 58 percent.

Study subjects: high-risk group with pre-diabetes
First degree relative of a type 2 diabetic
BMI >25
40–65 years old
pre-diabetic (impaired glucose tolerance)

Intervention group treatment

Goals: Participants were given specific goals and specific advice on how to achieve goals.

Strong intervention: Strong but infrequent intervention facilitated maintenance of physical health for at least 4 years.

Personalized: Dietary and exercise advice was given to each participant.

Diet:

- ≥ 5% weight reduction
- ≤ 30% fat intake
- ≤ 10% saturated fat intake
- Whole grains, vegetables, fruits, low-fat milk, low-fat meat, monounsaturated oils

Exercise program: The option for supervised, progressive, and individually tailored exercise programs were offered to participants. Participation rate was 50–85% at the various centers.

- ≥ 30' of moderate exercise daily was recommended.
- A personalized approach made a big difference.

Frequency: food records; 7 sessions with a nutritionist during the first year and quarterly in subsequent years.

NEJM study outcomes

- *Weight loss duration:* Intervention group kept the weight off significantly better than the control group for at least 4 years. A separate study demonstrates that intervention results and behaviors persist at least 7 years after the intervention was stopped (2).

- *Diet duration:* Diet recommendations made a difference in health maintenance for at least 4 years.

- *Exercise:* "It is likely that any type of physical activity—whether sports, household work, gardening, or work-related physical activity—is similarly beneficial in preventing diabetes."

- *Progression to diabetes:* The proportion of study subject who progressed to a diabetic state was twice as high in the non-intervention group.

- *Cumulative incidence of diabetes* was over twice as high in the non-intervention group. This incidence comparison was maintained at least 4 years after the beginning of the study.

- *Correlation of goal success with incidence of diabetes:* Diabetes did not develop in any of those who achieved 4 or 5 of the study goals. By contrast, diabetes developed in 38% of the intervention group who did not achieve any of their goals and 31% of the non-intervention group who did not achieve any of their goals.

- *Demanding program did not result in a high dropout rate:* "It is commonly argued that it is difficult to change the lifestyle of obese and sedentary people, but such pessimism may not be justified. The reasonably low dropout rate in our study also indicates that subjects with impaired glucose tolerance are willing and able to participate in a demanding intervention program if it is made available to them."

- *Overall conclusion by the researchers:* "This study provides evidence that type 2 diabetes can be prevented by changes in the lifestyles of both women and men at high risk for the disease. The overall incidence of diabetes was reduced by 58 percent."

1. Tuomilehto, J., et al. (2001). Prevention of type 2 diabetes mellitus by changes in lifestyle among subjects with impaired glucose tolerance. New England Journal of Medicine, 344(18): 1343-1350. doi:10.1056/NEJM200105033441801

2. Lindström, J., et al. (2006). Sustained reduction in the incidence of type 2 diabetes by lifestyle intervention: Follow-up of the Finnish diabetes prevention study. The Lancet, 368(9548), 1673-1679. http://dx.doi.org/10.1016/S0140-6736(06)69701-8

Summary of T2D prevention and reversal programs

A range of diets have effectively prevented or reversed diabetes. The question is not if there is one diet that prevents or reverses diabetes. The central questions appear to be:

- What are the core elements that should be included in every diet that is effective against diabetes?

- Which diet works best with the individual's genetic makeup, disease state, age, pocketbook, and other factors?

- Which studies need to be done to personalize diets and refine the core elements?

Core elements of the best modern diets

- Plant-based diet consisting of non-starchy vegetables and fruits

- Total plant component = 75%: Fresh plant-based foods make up about 75% of the total diet

- Very low levels (less than 10%) or elimination of simple carbohydrates

- 25–50% healthy fats (avocado, nuts, seeds, olive oil, coconut oil)

- Lean protein sources such as fish, chicken, poultry, and vegetable protein

- Long-term health community including a health coach

- Health monitoring and testing

- Consistent exercise at a moderate to vigorous level

Range of differences

Low fat versus high healthy fat
Grains versus no grains
Processed food versus non-processed food
Non-organic versus organic food
Dairy versus no dairy

Perspective on reversibility

In most people, T2D can be readily reversed if addressed. Perhaps even more encouraging is that T2D can be reversed in some very long-term patients if lifestyle changes are made. Even though the reversal process is more difficult with increased duration of the disease, it is very encouraging that advanced stages are not necessarily an obstacle. The degree of recovery difficulty is proportionate to the starting weight and duration. Thus, those who can address T2D early should do so, and many of those with an extended T2D duration can still recover. The main point

> Advanced stages of type 2 diabetes are not necessarily an obstacle to reversal.

is to not let T2D get to the point where major losses in beta cell function have occurred.

How to maintain reversibility

Maintaining reversibility is not difficult to understand. Unfortunately, simple processes can still be difficult to implement and maintain. A person who has achieved a T2D reversal simply needs to maintain the healthy lifestyle changes that helped them achieve reversal. The difficulty comes in resisting the constant temptation all of us have to return to the wrong foods and to not exercise. Planning, goals, and community can combine to maintain reversibility.

Planning: Set maintenance goals

Characteristics of maintenance goals

- *Margin:* An effective maintenance goal would provide a safety buffer to prevent any return to prediabetes or T2D. This will be person-specific. If you had to lose 50 pounds to achieve reversal, add a 10-pound margin. A 10-pound margin is in accordance with BMI boundaries.

- *Duration:* Because we learn and change with time, it is recommended that no more than annual goals are set.

- *Repetition:* Each year, review your progress and observe how your goals change as you learn and grow. It is recommended that a lifelong goal be set. Also set new maintenance goals every year for the rest of life. Why? If we stop the goal setting process, we will likely be manipulated by our feelings to return to unhealthy habits. Goals actually counteract the pressure put on us by our feelings and help us maintain gains in health.

- *Monitoring:* How often will you get tested for blood sugar, A1C, cholesterol, triglycerides, and any other parameters relevant to your situation? Annual testing is a minimum recommendation.

Exercise: Margin to prevent a return to T2D

How long do you want your goals to last? In the following table, put the goal duration in the left column for any goals you set. In the right-hand column, place the date you plan to review the goal. When you review it, you can reset it as is for the same duration, adjust it or replace it. When you finish a goal, record the date in the "Goal review and reset" section. If you find a plan that works well, you can set the goal duration as "indefinitely." The specifics are up to you.

Goal Duration and Repetition Table

Goal type	Goal duration	Goal review & reset
Nutrition		
Exercise		
Weight loss		
Community		
Monitoring		
Additional goal		
Additional goal		

Too many goals in the beginning can overcomplicate the recovery journey. Keep it to the basic elements that provided successful reversal and improve upon those. Once those habits become automatic, new goals can be added. Choose goals you can realistically achieve.

10
HOW TO LOSE WEIGHT AND KEEP IT OFF

THIS CHAPTER BEGINS with two stories to help people in their struggle to keep weight off. There are individuals that have to work much harder to maintain their health. Most people are not aware of the level of effort required to maintain a healthy weight or healthy lifestyle. Most are also not aware of their health status or the consequences of poor health. Because of this combination of factors, the percentage of those naturally prone to obesity who keep their weight at a healthy level is small. For those who do maintain their weight, their level of effort is very high. According to Kelly Brownell, director of the Rudd Center for Food Policy and Obesity at Yale University, "they never don't think about their weight" (1). Given this level of effort, foundational health is essential to weight loss success.

The National Weight Control Registry (2)

The National Weight Control Registry (NWCR) tracks 10,000 people who have lost weight and have kept it off. Kelly Brownell, director of the Rudd Center for Food Policy and Obesity at Yale University, stated that the 10,000 people tracked in the registry are a tiny percentage of the tens of millions of people who have tried unsuccessfully to lose weight.

Why NWCR was established: "We set it up in response to comments that nobody ever succeeds at weight loss," says Rena Wing, a professor of psychiatry and human behavior at Brown University's Alpert Medical School, who helped create the registry with James O. Hill, director of the Center for Human Nutrition at the University of Colorado at Denver.

NWCR goals: "We had two goals: to prove there were people who [succeed at weight loss], and to try to learn from them about what they do to achieve this long-term weight loss."

NWCR eligibility: Anyone who has lost 30 pounds and kept it off for at least a year is eligible to join the study.

NWCR results: The average member has lost 70 pounds and remained at that weight for six years.

Factors for weight regain: Wing indicated that she agrees that physiological changes probably do occur that make permanent weight loss difficult. She stated that the larger problem is environmental. People struggle to keep weight off because they are surrounded by food, inundated with food messages, and constantly presented with opportunities to eat. "We live in an environment with food cues all the time," Wing says. "We've taught ourselves over the years that one of the ways to reward yourself is with food. It's hard to change the environment and the behavior."

1. Parker-Pope, T. (2011, December). The fat trap. The New York Times Magazine. Retrieved from http://www.nytimes.com/2012/01/01/magazine/tara-parker-pope-fat-trap.html?pagewanted=all

2. The National Weight Control Registry. (n.d.). The National Weight Control Registry. Retrieved from http://www.nwcr.ws/

Question: How difficult is it for you to lose weight?

- Not difficult
- Somewhat difficult
- Very difficult
- Extremely difficult

How do people successfully maintain a healthy weight?	
NWCR	Weight Watchers, Jenny Craig, Atkins diet, surgery
Finnish Study	Intensive health coaching over an average 3 year period to establish healthy patterns (1)
Daniel Plan	Intensive community support in a long-term church environment combined with functional medicine diet (2)

1. Tuomilehto, J., et al. (2001). Prevention of type 2 diabetes mellitus by changes in lifestyle among subjects with impaired glucose tolerance. New England Journal of Medicine, 344(18): 1343-1350. doi:10.1056/NEJM200105033441801

2. Warren, R., Amen, D., & Hyman, M. (2013). The Daniel plan: 40 days to a healthier life. Grand Rapids, MI: Zondervan.

Some people have to work harder to keep weight off. Eating and exercise habits appear to reflect what researchers find in the lab: to lose weight and keep it off, a person must eat fewer calories and exercise far more than a person who maintains the same weight naturally. The following

> Some people have to work harder to keep weight off.

provides the metabolic basis of the higher level of effort required for a weight-reduced body and an example of the level of effort required to maintain weight loss in a weight-reduced body.

Metabolic basis of the higher level of effort required for a weight-reduced body (1)
Transformation to efficient slow twitch muscle fibers which burn less energy
Result of muscle transformation: After losing weight, your muscles burn 20 to 25 percent fewer calories during everyday activity

Metabolic basis: A weight-reduced body behaves differently from a similar-size body that has not dieted. "Muscle biopsies taken before, during and after weight loss show that once a person drops weight, their muscle fibers undergo a transformation, making them more like highly efficient 'slow twitch' muscle fibers. After losing weight, your muscles burn 20 to 25 percent fewer calories during everyday activity and moderate aerobic exercise than the muscles of a person who is naturally at the same weight. That means a dieter who thinks she is burning 200 calories during a brisk half-hour walk is probably using closer to 150 to 160 calories" (1).

Lower weight means eating fewer calories or cutting more carbs to stay at that weight. One woman who entered a Columbia University study at 230 pounds was eating about 3,000 calories to maintain that weight. Once she dropped to 190 pounds, losing 17 percent of her body weight, metabolic studies determined that she needed about 2,300 daily calories to maintain the new lower weight. A typical 30-year-old 190-pound woman can consume about 2,600 calories to maintain her weight. A woman who dieted to get to 190 pounds must eat 300 less calories per day than a woman who maintains that weight naturally (1).

1.   Parker-Pope, T. (2011, December). The fat trap. The New York Times Magazine. Retrieved from http://www.nytimes.com/2012/01/01/magazine/ tara-parker-pope-fat-trap.html?pagewanted=all

The URL below allows you to input your age, weight, and height while it calculates the calories you need to maintain your current weight and the calories needed to lose weight:

http://www.calculator.net/calorie-calculator.html

Substituting healthy fat (avocados, olive oil, nuts, and seeds) for starchy carbs and simple carbs can help a lot with this metabolic issue. This carb to healthy fat exchange adjusts your metabolism so you are not heavily penalized by your body for losing weight (1). Healthy fat and fiber allows you to feel full without a metabolic penalty from your body and does not require calorie counting. Quite a difference! On a high-carb diet, I have to exercise to prevent weight gain. On a high-fat, low-carb diet, I don't have to exercise to prevent weight gain.

Less entertainment: Those who keep the weight off watch less than half as much television as the overall population.

Diet discipline: Maintainers eat the same foods and in the same patterns consistently each day and don't "cheat" on weekends or holidays.

Calorie intake: They also appear to eat less than most people, with estimates ranging from 50 to 300 fewer daily calories.

Use the calorie burn calculator at http://www.healthstatus.com/perl/reload.pl to determine the level of exercise required for your goals.

1. Ludwig, D. (2016). Always hungry: Conquer cravings, retrain your fat cells, and lose weight permanently. New York, NY: Grand Central Publishing.

Janice's battle against regain (1)

Thought of food is always there. Janice is an NWCR member who has successfully maintained a 135-pound weight loss for about five years. According to Janice, maintaining weight loss is "one of the hardest things there is." "It's something that has to be focused on every minute. I'm not always thinking about food, but I am always aware of food."

Comfort eating: Janice and her husband each sought the help of therapists, and in her sessions, she learned that she had a tendency to eat when she was bored or stressed: "We are very much aware of how our culture taught us to use food for all kinds of reasons that aren't related to its nutritive value." "She avoids junk food, bread and pasta and many dairy products and tries to make sure nearly a third of her calories come from protein."

Hidden calories: "[They] will occasionally share a dessert, or eat an individual portion of Ben and Jerry's ice cream, so they know exactly how many calories they are ingesting. Because she knows errors can creep in, either because a rainy day cuts exercise short or a mismeasured snack portion adds hidden calories, she allows herself only 1,800 daily calories of food. (The average estimate for a similarly active woman of her age and size is about 2,300 calories.)"

The ease of regain: "It doesn't take a lot of variance from my current maintenance for me to pop on another two or three pounds," she says.

Weight Metrics and journaling: Since October 2006, Janice has weighed herself every morning and recorded the result in a weight diary. She even carries a scale with her when she travels. In the past six years, she made only one exception to this routine: a two-week, no-weigh vacation in Hawaii. Journaling "is really important; it's my accountability," she says. "It comes up with the total number of calories I've eaten today and the amount of protein. I do a little bit of self-analysis every night."

Exercise: "[Janice] supports her careful diet with an equally rigorous regimen of physical activity. She exercises from 100 to 120 minutes a day, six or seven days a week, often by riding her bicycle to the gym, where she takes a water-aerobics class. She also works out on an elliptical trainer at home and uses a recumbent bike to 'walk' the dog, who loves to run alongside the low, three-wheeled machine. She enjoys gardening as a hobby but allows herself to count it as exercise on only those occasions when she needs to 'garden vigorously.' Adam, her husband, is also a committed exerciser, riding his bike at least two hours a day, five days a week."

Metabolism: Based on metabolic data Janice "collected from the weight-loss clinic and her own calculations, she has discovered that to keep her current weight of 195 pounds, she can eat 2,000 calories a day as long as she burns 500 calories in exercise."

Schedule: "Just talking to [Janice] about the effort required to maintain her weight is exhausting. [Janice] concedes that having grown children and being retired make it easier to focus on her weight. 'I don't know if I could have done this when I had three kids living at home,' she says. 'We know how unusual we are. It's pretty easy to get angry with the amount of work and dedication it takes to keep this weight off. But the alternative is to not keep the weight off.'"

Is it worth it?

The high level of effort is worth it. "It's been a real struggle to stay at this weight, but it's worth it, it's good for me, it makes me feel better. But my body would put on weight almost instantaneously if I ever let up." "So she never lets up."

For many overweight people who still try to lose weight with low fat, high carb diets, there are probably easier ways to lose weight. Even when people cut back on carbs, they may eat too many other starchy foods like potatoes. If 90–100% of starchy carbs are replaced with healthy fat, protein and fiber, metabolism can be adjusted significantly. Fat consumption speeds up metabolism. Most people don't cut out enough starchy carbs, which keeps them in the metabolic penalty zone.

How much time and energy can people save on a low carb diet?

- **Enormous thought energy:** healthy fat and fiber reduce cravings.

- **Exercise time:** 25-50% healthy fat and removal of refined carbohydrates facilitates weight loss without exercise. Exercise time can also be reduced by interval training.

- **Calorie counting time:** Functional medicine diets are designed to eliminate the need for calorie counting.

Why recovery is needed

> When starchy carbs are eliminated, so are cravings

Food addiction: "The body, in order to get back to its pre-diet weight, induces cravings by making the person feel more excited about food and giving him or her less willpower to resist a high-calorie treat" (1). Cravings are another penalty of keeping too many starchy or simple carbs in the diet. Cravings won't change as long as starchy carbs are still there. When starchy carbs are eliminated, so are cravings (2). Each person can determine what level of starchy carbs stimulates cravings by eliminating them and adding them back.

> **Changes in the brain after weight loss if starchy carbs are still in the diet**

When a dieter looked at food	bigger response in the parts of the brain associated with reward
	lower response in the areas associated with eating restraint
	greater emotional response to food
	Dieters want food more
Duration of brain's defense of the higher weight	6 years

1. Parker-Pope, T. (2011, December). The fat trap. The New York Times Magazine. Retrieved from http://www.nytimes.com/2012/01/01/magazine/tara-parker-pope-fat-trap.html?pagewanted=all

2. Hyman, M. (n.d.). 10 day detox diet starter kit. Retrieved from http://www.10daydetoxcookbook.com/?a_aid=54ef3e65242a0&a_bid=944fd4dd&chan=code4

Exercise: Foundational health to keep the weight off

1. In what areas of weight loss do you need the most help?

____

____

____

____

2. What is the importance of your weight loss community to your journey toward health? How can they support your journey and help you maintain health?

____

____

____

____

____

3. If your struggle is in a different area of health, what areas do you need the most help with and how can your recovery community help you?

____

____

____

____

____

4. How many starchy or simple carbs do you eat per day?

____

____

____

____

____

Exercise: Wellness Screening

Go over the results of the test in chapter 8 with your doctor.

- Is your glucose level in a normal range?
- Does a normal range mean that no damage has been done?
- How often do you plan to monitor blood glucose?
- What boundaries can you set with weight, diet, and exercise to give yourself margin against pancreatic damage? When do you plan to start working toward your buffer goal?

Weight loss is much harder for some people because of metabolic variance. Thus, some may prefer to set goals based on a combination of feeling better and achieving a reasonable standard of health. For those with good genetics, they can tolerate some level excess weight. Unfortunately, some will not have the genetics needed to tolerate excess weight. If your family history includes a high incidence of diabetes or heart disease, excess weight will not likely be tolerated well by your body.

In setting weight boundaries, consider the following: In a BMI table, several weight ranges are considered normal below the first range that is considered overweight. Do you want to do more than make it into the highest weight category within the normal range? Why not give yourself margin and go one category below? For example, a normal BMI range for a person who is 5' 9" starts at a BMI score of 18 and peaks at 24. A BMI of 25 is the first BMI score that is considered overweight. Reaching a BMI of 25 provides no extra buffer. A BMI score of 24 would provide a 5-pound buffer.

A minimum exercise recommendation to stay in the healthy range is 30' per day. A buffer range would add extra exercise minutes such as 45–60 minutes. Buffer ranges for diet can be added in accordance with the healthy diet you choose. For example, you could cut the number of servings of carbohydrates below that recommended by your diet to give yourself some buffer.

Buffers against organ and cell damage			
Parameter	Healthy range	Buffer range	Start date
Weight (BMI score)			
Diet program			
Exercise (minutes/day)			

Many people can maintain a relatively healthy lifestyle and remain somewhat overweight if they eat a healthy diet, exercise regularly, and engage in holistic health. However, there is no guarantee. It is your decision as to how much risk you want to take with your health. The more margin you give yourself by losing weight below the overweight range, the greater your chances of consistently high-level health.

In addition to analyzing your current risk, it is also useful to understand your future risk for T2D. The ADA's My Health Advisor calculates your 8-year risk for diabetes, stroke, and heart disease. People with type 2 diabetes are at increased risk for stroke and heart disease. Thus, it is important to assess risk for stroke and heart disease as well.

Exercise: Risk for diabetes, stroke, and heart disease

- Determine your future risk for diabetes, stroke, and heart disease using ADA's My Health Advisor. http://main.diabetes.org/dorg/mha/main_en_US.html?loc=dorg-mha

- How can you use this information to better your health? Do the results reinforce or add to your response to the diabetes risk test?

Exercise: Measuring Belly Fat

The location of excess fat on the body is important. A waist measurement of 40 inches or more for men and 35 inches or more for women is linked to insulin resistance and increases a person's risk for type 2 diabetes. This linkage is true even if a person's BMI falls within the normal range (1). Removing belly fat through weight loss is challenging because belly fat can remain over the recommended levels even after we lose significant weight. Essentially, belly fat can help gauge buffer weight loss because it often doesn't come off completely until we are well within the normal weight range. If we lose the belly fat through exercise and nutrition, we've probably created our first significant weight buffer.

Measure your belly fat

1. Measure your belly fat according to the instructions below and record here
2. What weight loss goal would bring your waist measurement into the safe range?

How to Measure the Waist

To measure the waist, a person should:

- Place a tape measure around the bare abdomen just above the hip bone
- Make sure the tape is snug but isn't digging into the skin and is parallel to the floor
- Relax, exhale, and measure
- National Institute of Diabetes and Digestive and Kidney Diseases. (n.d.). Overweight & obesity statistics. Retrieved from https://www.niddk.nih.gov/health-information/health-statistics/Pages/overweight-obesity-statistics.aspx

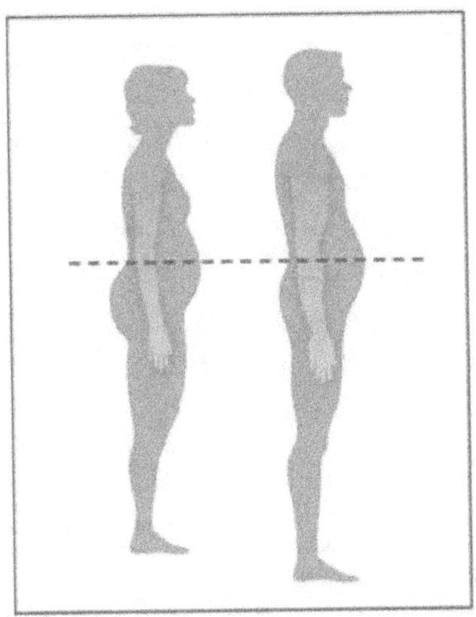

Weight loss goals

BMI

BMI is a simple and effective self-measure that quickly reveals important health information for individuals or communities. BMI is an inexpensive and easy-to-perform method of screening for weight.

What is BMI?

According to the CDC, "Body Mass Index (BMI) is a number calculated from a person's weight and height. BMI is a fairly reliable indicator of body fatness for most people. BMI does not measure body fat directly, but research has shown that BMI correlates to direct measures of body fat, such as underwater weighing and dual energy x-ray absorptiometry (DXA)" (1).

Why is BMI used?

There is no need for expensive techniques in most cases. BMI saves time and money while providing valuable screening information. According to the CDC, "Calculating BMI is one of the best methods for population assessment of overweight and obesity. Because calculation requires only height and weight, it is inexpensive and easy to use for clinicians and for the general public."

BMI	Weight Status
Below 18.5	Underweight
18.5–24.9	Normal
25.0–29.9	Overweight
30.0 and Above	Obese

Centers for Disease Control and Prevention. (2015). About adult BMI. Retrieved from http://www.cdc.gov/healthyweight/assessing/bmi/adult_bmi/

Potential for improvement

Potential weight loss improvements: Extreme obesity is a category that is growing faster than any other (1). Consider the following example for American men of average height in terms of the potential weight loss required to return to normal weight:

Over 400 lbs: >58% body weight loss needed
Over 300 lbs: >44% body weight loss needed
Over 200 lbs: >16% body weight loss needed

Consider if the 5% weight loss recommendation by some health programs for a person of average height were interpreted the same by every dieter. If persons with extreme obesity fol-lowed the 5% recommendation, they would not likely achieve the health outcomes they desire.

	5% body weight loss	Weight loss required to return to recommended weight	
	lbs	% body weight	lbs
Over 400 lbs	20	>58%	232
Over 300 lbs	15	>44%	132
Over 200 lbs	10	>16%	32

If a person has extreme obesity, a low standard goal of 5% is insufficient to return them to health. A 15 lb loss for a 300-pound person of average height will leave them in poor health and at risk for problems associated with heart disease and T2D. The NIH DPP studies showed that significant health improvement can be obtained with a 5% weight loss for a 200 lb person of average height. In order to return to their recommended weight, a 400 lb person of average height needs to lose about 200 pounds, 10 times the 5% level. The more obese a person is, the more weight they will need to lose in order to get into the healthy range. The BMI guidelines are a simple and clear guideline for determining the amount of weight that needs to be lost. Exceptions include athletes with a large amount of muscle mass.

1. National Institute of Diabetes and Digestive and Kidney Diseases. (n.d.). Overweight & obesity statistics. Retrieved from https://www.niddk.nih.gov/health-information/health-statistics/Pages/overweight-obesity-statistics.aspx

BMI calculator

http://www.nhlbi.nih.gov/health/educational/lose_wt/BMI/
bmicalc.htm

Exercise: Calculation of weight loss goal

1. Using your height, determine your health weight range from the BMI table or calculator.

2. If you are overweight, subtract a recommended weight within the healthy range of the BMI table from your weight to determine your weight loss goal.

Exercise: Fitness plan

A number of different systems have proven to be effective in addressing physical health long term. There is never any guarantee in the program itself. It depends on the willingness of the participant to engage the program. More importantly, lifelong fitness depends on a lifelong commitment to fitness.

Self-motivated people maintain their physical fitness, whether or not they participate in a program. Most people who are not physically fit need a program to get them started on the right track. Sports put me on the right track in grade school. I have never stopped exercising except for injury, but there was a 2–3-year period when I was not physically fit. My lack of fitness spiritually, mentally, and emotionally had begun to affect my physical health. I was nearly obese at one point. My fitness plan needed a greater emphasis in the non-physical foundational areas of health.

1. Choose a holistic, community-oriented fitness plan with demonstrated, long-term results.

2. Review your progress after 6 months. At that time, ask what improvements have occurred and how much improvement is still needed to reach your weight goal.

3. Self-evaluate again after 6 months. Are there new priorities? If so, search for programs that can help you with the new priority.

4. Complete a wellness profile blood screening at a local clinic and review the Physical Health Decision Table below to determine the health level of your weight loss goal. If you are helping someone else lose weight, discuss the decision table with them.

Question: What are your thoughts on choosing a weight goal?

Healthy weight loss goals

A standard blood profile to determine cholesterol levels, blood sugar levels, and other indicators is an effective tool for monitoring physical health. In distinguishing the difference between a healthy goal and an unhealthy goal, consider the following Physical Health Evaluation Table:

Physical Health Evaluation Table			
Condition/state	Healthy	Inter-mediate	Unhealthy
Healthy wellness profile/ healthy weight	x		
Healthy weight/ wellness profile warnings		x	

Overweight/ wellness profile warnings		x	x
Obese/ wellness profile warnings			x

Intermediate states of health are problematic because they leave the individual vulnerable to conditions such as T2D. The following conclusions from a research study clarify that:

The more weight a person loses, the greater their chances of reversing T2D.

The longer a person has T2D, the less chance they have of reversing T2D (1).

To minimize chances of T2D, a person needs to reach and maintain their recommended weight by eating healthy food.

Study Summary (Steven S., et al., 2013)

Those who quickly engaged in a reversal program and lost a significant amount of weight were at least twice as likely to reverse diabetes as those who did not.

A study by Steven et al. (1) examined diabetes reversal at different levels of weight loss and after different durations of diabetes. "Diabetes reversal was considered to have occurred in 61% of the population. Reversal of diabetes was observed in 80, 63 and 53% of those with > 20, 10–20 and < 10 kg weight loss, respectively. There was a significant correlation between degree of weight loss and reported fasting glucose levels (Rs -0.38, P = 0.006)." Reversal rates according to diabetes duration were:

Weight Loss	Reversal Rate	Duration of T2D	Reversal Rate
>20 kg/44 lb	80%	< 4 years	73%
10-20 kg/ 22–44 lb	63%	4–8 years	56%
< 10 kg/ 22 lb	53%	> 8 years	43%

Web MD recommends ways that those with morbid obesity lose at least 100 lb (2).

1. Steven, S., Lim, E. L., & Taylor, R. (2013). Population response to information on reversibility of type 2 diabetes. Diabetic Medicine, 30(4), e135-e138. doi:10.1111/dme.12116

2. WebMD. (2015). Tips to lose 100 pounds or more. Retrieved from http://www.webmd.com/diet/features/10 -tips-losing-100-pounds-or-more

11

T2D REVERSAL PROCESS

Advantages of healthy fat

High-carb, low-fat food pyramids are perhaps the worst nutritional guidelines in history.

SINCE THE 1970s, both the scientific community and the general public believed the prevailing nutritional science that all fat was bad and that all calories are created equal. Why? Because funding for scientifically sound nutritional studies was not forthcoming in a treatment-oriented culture. It followed that low-fat, high-carbohydrate diets were considered healthy. Unfortunately, low-fat, high-carb diets have been a major determinant of the obesity and type 2 diabetes epidemics. These diets are also a major determinant of why so many people have struggled to lose weight. High-carb, low-fat food pyramids are perhaps the worst nutritional guidelines in history.

According to David Ludwig, Harvard endocrinologist, low-fat, high-carbohydrate diets program our fat cells to "hoard too many calories leaving too few for the rest of the body" (1). In other words, our body thinks we are starving. As a result, hunger persists, metabolism slows, and weight is gained. In an effort to lose weight, people cut calories, which actually makes things worse, by initiating a never-ending and unnecessary battle between mind and body. We literally fight ourselves under these conditions. Weight gain is driven by insulin which stimulates fat cells to take up blood glucose and store it as fat. Carbs are the most powerful stimulant of insulin production. Fat affects insulin production the least. Thus, if we want to reduce fat storage and lose weight, we need to eat much more healthy fat and much less carbohydrate.

Our high-carb diets have been stimulating the overproduction of insulin. A barrage of insulin spikes occurs daily because of the frequent consumption of refined carbohydrates by the vast majority of Americans. This barrage eventually damages our cells and contributes to insulin resistance, a major risk factor for heart disease. To further complicate matters, sugar slows our metabolism, an undesirable effect for losing weight. In contrast, fat increases our metabolism. The main risk factors for heart disease are insulin resistance, diabetes, high blood pressure, smoking, previous history of heart conditions, excess weight, belly fat circumference, high triglycerides, and low HDLs. Almost all of these risk factors can be dramatically improved by reducing carbs and increasing healthy fats. Deprivation won't work. Healthy fat does work. Functional medicine diets allow you to eat until satisfied and never count calories again. If you eat in accordance with the natural design of your metabolism, your body will do the rest.

When someone begins diabetes reversal, exercise is optional for those too unhealthy for exercise. Some individuals are unable to exercise at their starting point because of body size and health complications. Low-carb, high healthy fat diets can help these individuals achieve very significant weight loss and get to a point where exercise is possible.

> Most heart disease risk factors can be dramatically improved by reducing carbs and increasing healthy fats.

To summarize, fat is healthy, and it helps us lose weight because (1,2):

- Fat reprograms our fat cells by reducing the production of insulin.

- Reprogrammed fat cells release calories back into the body to be burned instead of stored.

- Fat increases our metabolism.

- Healthy fat leads to higher levels of HDL cholesterol and better cholesterol ratios.

- Healthy fat reduces risk of both diabetes and heart disease.

1. Ludwig, D. (n.d.). Take back control. David Ludwig MD PHD. Retrieved from https://www.drdavidludwig.com/

2. Hyman, M. (2016). Eat fat, get thin: Why the fat we eat is the key to sustained weight loss and vibrant health. New York, NY: Little, Brown and Company.

Weight control through healthy fat

High carb weight gain: I had a bike accident in 2001. I was riding back to the train station at night with my head down to keep the sleet and rain out of my face while I sped down a hill. I don't remember anything else after this point other than what I was told. I woke up in the hospital in the middle of the night. My jacket and clothes had been cut off me. I fractured a rib or 2 and my collarbone, injured my ankle, cracked my helmet completely through, and bent my bike frame.

I was unable to exercise because of my injuries for a couple of months as the fractures healed. As a result, I gained about 20 pounds for the first time in my life. I had never gained weight, so I didn't expect it. I was completely surprised. At that time, I was still on a high-carb diet following the USDA food pyramid. Carbs accounted for probably 75–95% of my caloric intake. Many days, I ate essentially 100% carbs (cereal for breakfast and supper; pasta for lunch), thinking that was healthy.

Healthy fat/fiber weight control: Fast forward to a chronic knee injury in 2015. For the previous year and a half, I had engaged in a high-incline, high-intensity treadmill regime. However, this program greatly aggravated my problem left knee. Eventually, my knee would flare up any time I did any kind of exercise. It took about six months of trying several different stretches and activity patterns suggested by doctors before it began to resolve. I didn't exercise for about 4 months during that period. I tried to restart exercise several times, and my knee flared up every time. My inactivity period was about 2 months longer than the bike accident, but I only gained 2–3 pounds. This small gain came off within a few days after resuming exercise. My high healthy fat diet, including lots of non-starchy vegetables, made the difference.

Question: How have carbs affected you?

Impact of calories:

- The amount of calories consumed impacts how much activity is needed.
- The type of calories consumed impacts how easy it is to lose weight and maintain weight loss.

Cutting calories below normal intake levels is not necessary if a functional medicine diet is consumed. Exercise is very important for health and decreasing insulin resistance. It is not required for weight loss, even though it helps.

It is best to start weight loss with a detox diet that controls cravings through fat and fiber. Craving control will vary with the individual. My cravings changed within 4 days on the Hyman detox (1).

Detox Phase

- Objectives
  - Craving control
  - Weight loss
  - Momentum for longer-term diet change
- Timing: First stage
- Duration: 10 days
- Off limits foods. No exceptions for 10 days
  - Sugar and all sweeteners (natural and artificial)
  - Gluten
  - Dairy
  - Grains
  - Beans
  - All processed foods
  - All simple carbohydrates

After completing the detox, the following tips for daily craving control are suggested (2):

- Eat a small meal or snack that includes healthy protein, like seeds or nuts, every 3 to 4 hours.

- Eliminate liquid calories and artificial sweeteners. "Try sticking with water and green tea. Green tea contains plant chemicals that are good for your health. And, last but not least, don't succumb to the diet-drink trap. The artificial sweeteners in diet drinks fool the body into thinking it is ingesting sugar, which creates the same insulin spike as regular sugar."

- Eat a high-quality protein at breakfast. Every meal should include high-quality protein, but it is especially important at breakfast. Studies show that waking up to a healthy protein, such as eggs, nuts, seeds, nut butters, or a protein shake help people lose weight, reduce cravings, and burn calories.

1. Hyman, M. (n.d.). 10 day detox diet starter kit. Retrieved from http://www.10daydetoxcookbook.com/?a_aid=54ef3e65242a0&a_bid=944fd4dd&chan=code4

2. Hyman, M. (n.d.). How to rewire your brain to end food cravings. Dr. Hyman. Retrieved from http://drhyman.com/blog/2012/03/01/how-to-rewire-your-brain-to-end-food-cravings/

Resetting our fat cells deals with cravings

Dr. David Ludwig, MD, Ph.D., is an influential researcher at Harvard. He has been one of the main voices who have clarified what is fundamentally wrong with low-fat, high-carb diets. His research team and other colleagues have been the ones gathering the data on what's amiss with low-fat consumption.

Because of their work, we now understand why dieting that works is not about eating less. It's about what you eat.

Dr. Ludwig and others have figured out how to calm fat cells down by reprogramming them. Insulin stimulates fat cells to take up calories from the blood. Carbohydrate is what stimulates the most insulin production. Too much insulin leads to too much weight stored in the fat cells. When this happens, we can't fight our fat cells because they are in hoarding mode. Our metabolism is misaligned under these conditions.

To realign our metabolism, we need to reprogram the fat cells by eating more fat. Once we start on a diet that takes care of our cravings through this reprogramming process, we're able to achieve a lower body weight set point. The new set point is established at a lower weight when you eat healthy fat. According to Dr. Ludwig, it takes about a month to reset our metabolism (1).

1. Ludwig, D. (2016). Always hungry: Conquer cravings, retrain your fat cells, and lose weight permanently. New York, NY: Grand Central Publishing.

Exercise: Quiz to determine if you are eating enough healthy fat

Take the quiz at the URL listed below and answer the following questions:

http://drhyman.com/blog/q/are-you-getting-enough-fat-quiz/

Question: How much healthy fat is in your diet? Are you eating enough?

Question: What foods could you eat more of?

What sources of fat should you include in your diet?

2015 marked a major turning point for dietary cholesterol recommendations. For decades, Americans heard the recommendations advising decreased intake of cholesterol from food sources such as butter and eggs and other high-fat foods. In an about-face, the dietary guidelines changed in 2015 to consider dietary cholesterol as an issue no longer of significant concern (1).

This change occurred because of the overwhelming evidence in support of healthy fat as part of a healthy diet (2). Healthy fat diets are being used to help thousands of people reverse diabetes by getting insulin production under control (3).

Which fats are healthy?

- Avocado
- Nuts and seeds
- Olive oil
- Fish oil
- Sardines
- Salmon

The above is a list of good sources of healthy fat. Fish oil is an excellent source of omega-3 fats and the best way to reduce inflammation. Reduced inflammation, in turn, is a major component of addressing several different types of chronic disease.

1. U.S. Department of Agriculture. (2015). Dietary guidelines for Americans: 2015-2020 (8th ed.). Retrieved from https://health.gov/dietaryguidelines/2015/resources/2015-2020_Dietary_Guidelines.pdf

2. Ludwig, D. (2016). Always hungry: Conquer cravings, retrain your fat cells, and lose weight permanently. New York, NY: Grand Central Publishing.

3. Hyman, M. (2016). Eat fat, get thin: Why the fat we eat is the key to sustained weight loss and vibrant health. New York, NY: Little, Brown and Company.

Reversal Phase

Importance of fiber in diabetes reversal

After the detox phase, you will have gained momentum for the reversal phase. Fiber is an important part of diabetes reversal. It helps prevent and reverse T2D by slowing the rate at which food enters your bloodstream and increasing the speed at which food exits your body through the digestive tract. Advantages of fiber also include:

- Balances your blood sugar and cholesterol
  - fiber can lower blood sugar as effectively as some diabetic medication
- Quickly eliminates toxins from your gut
- Reduces your appetite and promotes weight loss
- Provides food for the healthy bacteria that promote health
- Natural cure for constipation and irregularity
- Can eliminate the need for insulin
- Reduces the risk of colon cancer by as much as a third and breast cancer by almost 40%
- Lowers cholesterol and reduces the risk of heart disease by as much as 40%

Dr. Denis Burkitt studied the importance of fiber by examining the differences between indigenous African Bushmen and their "civilized" western counterparts. "The Bushmen seemed to be free of the scourges of modern life including heart disease, cancer, diabetes and obesity." He discovered large differences in fiber consumption. The average American eats about 8 to 15 grams of fiber a day; the average hunter-gatherer ate 100 to 150 grams of a variety of roots, berries, leaves, and plant foods (1).

The bacteria in your gut metabolize soluble fiber from fruits, vegetables, beans, nuts, seeds, and most whole grains. This leads to lower cholesterol, blood sugar, and insulin, cancer prevention, balanced hormone levels, and production of vital vitamins and minerals.

Glucomannan (GM), a soluble, fermentable and highly viscous dietary fiber that helps you lose weight, lowers your cholesterol, reduces your appetite, and lowers your blood sugar more effectively than any other fiber. It is derived from the root of the Asian elephant yam, also known as konjac. "It can absorb up to 50 times its weight in water, making it one of the most viscous dietary fibers known" (1). Glucomannan works by promoting a sense of fullness. The fiber pushes more calories out through your colon, rather than letting them be absorbed.

How does glucomannan promote weight loss (1)?

- GM lowers the energy density of the food you eat. It bulks up food in your gut, creating a lower calorie content per weight of food you eat. Since fiber has almost no calories but a lot of weight, adding it to the diet lowers the energy-to-weight ratio of the food that is consumed.

- o Studies show that it is the volume or weight of food that controls our appetite. The GM fiber increases the weight WITHOUT increasing calories.
- GM can signal the brain that there is a lot of food in our gut, sending the message to slow down eating. It moves through the stomach and the small bowel slowly because it is so viscous.
  - o By slowing the rate of food absorption from the gut to the bloodstream, it reduces the amount of insulin produced after a meal. This insulin reduction lowers your appetite.
- More energy (calories) is lost through the stool because the calories are all soaked into the fiber.

Options for increasing daily fiber (1)

30 to 50 grams a day:

- 2 tablespoons of ground flax seeds a day added to your food.
- Beans can be included if you can tolerate them (all forms of legumes).
- Large quantities of vegetables – with almost no calories, high levels of antioxidants, and protective phytochemicals, are excellent fiber sources.
- Whole grains like brown rice or quinoa can be added if you can tolerate them.
- A few servings of low-sugar fruits can be added to your diet daily (berries are the highest in fiber and other protective phytochemical).

- Almonds, walnuts, pecans, or hazelnuts and seeds like pumpkin, chia, and hemp can be added to your diet every day.

- 2 to 4 capsules of PGX (Natural Factors) can be consumed with a glass of water before eating. Or take 2.5 to 5 grams of the powder form. Make sure you drink plenty of water throughout the day when taking PGX, as you can become constipated.

1. Hyman, M. (n.d.). How to eat 12 pounds of food and lose weight. Dr. Hyman. Retrieved from http://drhyman.com/blog/2016/09/01/how-to-eat-12-pounds-of-food-and-lose-weight/

How do you personalize your diet?

The best diet is the one optimized to your individual biology. Functional medicine helps accomplish this through testing. The following tests fine tune your diet to your specific genetics:

- Food sensitivity testing

- Food allergy testing

- Genetic testing: genetic predisposition to cardiovascular risk, obesity, cancer, or other conditions relevant to diet

- Wellness profiles (cholesterol, blood sugar, triglycerides, blood pressure)

Analyses in randomized trials showed that genetic markers for obesity, diabetes, or cardiovascular disease might modify the metabolic response to weight-loss diets. Genetic predisposition to cardiovascular risk or obesity can also be modified by dietary patterns or consumption of sugar-sweetened beverages (1). More well-designed studies on gene-diet interactions are under way. Diet studies demonstrate considerable genetic heterogeneity in a variety of metabolic functions in response to diet interventions (1). The findings support personalized interventions according to individual genotype.

1. Qi, L. (2012). Gene-diet interactions in complex diseases: Current findings and relevance for public health. Current Nutrition Reports, 1(4), 222-227. doi:10.1007/s13668-012-0029-8

JETT PHC's Living in Reverse program is based on the foundation of functional medicine.

The main tenets are as follows (1):

Remove or replace simple carbohydrates: High carb consumption creates high insulin levels, eventually leading to insulin resistance and type 2 diabetes. The most important factor in reducing the risk of type 2 diabetes and obesity or reversing their impact is to eliminate or dramatically reduce sugar in all forms.

Whole, unprocessed foods: Whole, unprocessed foods balance your blood sugar, reduce inflammation and oxidative stress, and improve your liver detoxification to prevent or reverse insulin resistance and diabetes. Choose a rich variety of colorful fruits and vegetables, plenty of omega-3 fats, coconut butter and olive oil, legumes, nuts, and seeds. The advantages of whole, real foods include:

- Whole foods turn on all the right gene messages
- Whole foods promote a healthy metabolism
- Whole foods reverse insulin resistance and diabetes
- Whole foods prevent aging and age-related diseases like diabetes and heart disease

Helpful nutrients: Supplements make your cells more sensitive to insulin and more effective at metabolizing sugar and fat. The following list of supplements is a good starting point (1):

- A high-quality multivitamin and mineral
- One to two grams of omega 3 fatty acids
- 1,000–2,000 IUs of vitamin D3
- 300–600 mg of alpha lipoic acid twice daily
- 200–600 mcg of chromium polynicotinate
- 2.5 to 5 grams of PGX, a unique type of fiber that controls appetite and blood sugar, before each meal with eight ounces of water

1. Hyman, M. (2014, December 18). 7 Steps to Reverse Obesity and Diabetes [Web log post]. Retrieved from http://drhyman.com/blog/2014/12/1 8/7-ways-reverse-obesity-diabetes/

Exercise: Consistent exercise of various types is key to reducing insulin resistance. Vigorous exercise is the key to balancing blood sugar and lowering insulin levels. Get your heart rate up to 70–80% of its maximum capacity for 60 minutes, up to six times a week. High-intensity interval training (HIIT) and strength training can be done in just minutes a day.

Get sufficient sleep: "Lack of sleep or poor sleep damages your metabolism, spikes sugar and carb cravings, makes you eat more, and increases your risk for numerous diseases including type 2 diabetes. One study among healthy subjects found even a partial night's poor sleep could induce insulin resistance." You must prioritize sleep so you get eight hours of solid sleep every night.

Control stress levels: Insulin, cortisol, and inflammatory compounds all increase in response to chronic stress. "This drives the relentless metabolic dysfunction that leads to weight gain, insulin resistance, and eventually type 2 diabetes. The links between stress, weight gain, mental disorders, and blood sugar imbalances show that managing stress becomes a critical component of obesity and diabetes management." Learning to control stress is essential to health. Stress can be controlled through meditation; deep breathing exercises, yoga, massage, laughing, and dancing are among the best ways to manage stress and reverse type 2 diabetes.

Measure to improve: Research shows that people who track their results lose twice as much weight. Begin by getting a journal to track your progress. Record a baseline of all measurements: your weight, waist size, body mass index (BMI), and blood pressure (optional). "Many patients become inspired when they see their results on paper."

1.   Hyman, M. (n.d.). 7 steps to reverse obesity and diabetes. Dr. Hyman. Retrieved from http://drhyman. com/blog/2014/12/18/7-ways-reverse-obesity-diabetes/

Living in Reverse Health Coaching Program

The purpose of the first section, What Causes T2D, is to help participants understand what contributes to T2D so they know what to stop doing. The middle section engages participants in a process based on functional medicine. Functional medicine programs have helped thousands of people reverse early stage T2D, pre-diabetes and other diet-driven chronic diseases (1). The final section helps participants help others improve their wellness by teaching and coaching others through the same steps that helped improve their own health. This process of passing along lessons reinforces those lessons in the participant's own recovery. Living in Reverse is found at www.jettphc.com.

Contact me for more information at tschierer@jettphc.com.

Living in Reverse health coaching program is divided into 3 sections:

- Chapters 1–3: The beginning section is designed to clarify the strong relationship between diet and type 2 diabetes. Once we know what the problem is, we can address it.

- Chapters 4–11: The middle section engages participants in a health recovery process based on functional medicine.

- Chapters 12–19: The final section covers wellness outreach. Helping others is the most powerful way we can reinforce our own recovery.

1. Hyman, Mark. Blood Sugar Solution. New york, NY, Little, Brown and Company, 2014.

12

PHYSICAL AND NON-PHYSICAL HEALTH INVENTORIES

How to identify health concerns in any area

THERE ARE 7 known areas of health. Physical health, vocational health, and financial health are based on the foundation of spiritual, relational, emotional health, and mental health. Programs emphasizing physical wellness alone are insufficient to ensure long-term health. Insufficient program duration also impacts effectiveness. Programs lasting at least one year and including health coaches and workout partners tend to be the most effective. Programs lasting 3 years or more create enough momentum that participants tend to maintain lifelong wellness behaviors (1). Recovery-oriented health programs continue indefinitely. Short-term programs are important steps in the growth journey, but recovery requires lifelong learning and growth. Living in Reverse combines the advantages of a recovery approach with the advantages of professional health coaching.

1. Tuomilehto , J. (2001). Prevention of type 2 diabetes mellitus by changes in lifestyle among subjects with impaired glucose tolerance. *N Engl J Med,344,* 1343-1350. doi:10.1056/NEJM200105033441801

Advantages of a recovery approach to health
Effective
Long-term
Programs accessible in every major city domestically and many international cities
Long-term reduction in medical and prescription costs
Holistic
Recovery is self-reinforced through helping others
Comprehensive

Recovery is comprehensive, normal, and practical

Recovery works because it is comprehensive. 12 step recovery programs have generated the highest levels of personal maturity, happiness, and resilience possible because of the comprehensive *nature* of the recovery process. The 12 steps are what *any* person implements in becoming to mature, regardless of whether they have ever participated in a 12-step program. For example, successful marriages are characterized by the 12 steps, regardless of whether either partner has participated in a 12-step program. Marriage is the most common place where people learn how to focus on their own faults and not the faults of another person. The nature of relationships requires this mindset. Relationships don't work in the absence of the ability to let go of the faults of others because resentment blocks our ability to be authentic and vulnerable. People acquire recovery relationship skills by handling resentments in a healthy way internally. Recovery helps us see our part in any situation and focus on that part only, undistracted by what happens to us or by what others do to us. This seemingly impossible perspective becomes possible when we realize that we give ourselves emotional health when we treat others as we want to be treated. The opposite is also true. If we are treated poorly and respond with negative behavior, it damages our emotional health.

Recovery is a powerful process that people with successful relationships have been practicing throughout history. It is nothing new. The naming of the process has changed over time, but the process has not changed. Some of those who have never been through a 12-step program are repulsed at the notion of participating in a recovery group. However, if they have successful relationships free of resentment, they have already been practicing the 12 steps, whether they realize it or not. Participants in this program do not have to identify themselves as recovery participants. This is not a dedicated 12-step program, but it is a program that incorporates recovery principles and steps. It is my hope that participants will understand their participation in this health recovery program as a normal process that may already be part of their life. As such, any discomfort associated with recovery terminology can dissipate.

Recovery is a process that can work under any circumstance. If we are feeling bad about ourselves in response to something that has happened to us, it means that we are judging ourselves as a result of what happened to us. If we are judging ourselves, something is wrong with our attitudes because we are no longer in a mindset of unconditional love. *By nature,* no external can *make us* feel bad. Instead, what is going on is a failure to accept ourselves. We wrong others by holding onto resentments. However, resentments harm us far more.

Usually, resentments do not harm others because the people we resent may not be aware that they offended us.

Recovery works under harsh conditions because it helps us understand that something is wrong with us if we judge ourselves in any way by what happens to us. The ultimate self-affirmation of our identity is unconditional self-love when we are treated poorly. When people begin to experience the power of this type of self-affirmation, it creates a healthy [addiction] to personal growth, seeing difficulties as opportunities for self-affirmation and an opportunity to change oneself for the better. It is a real process. People experience this power and freedom over circumstances and want more of it.

- Recovery is internal
- Recovery is identity-based
- Recovery is practical
    - Centered around what we can do for ourselves
- Recovery is a normal part of successful relationships
- Recovery is a process

Recovery is a process of complete surrender in which we give up our reliance on externals to secure our identity. It is a decision to accept ourselves unconditionally under any circumstance through our belief and reliance on unconditional self-love, unconditional love from our Creator, or both. Professional coaching and the 12 steps of recovery have the same personal identity foundation: Unconditional self-love through a higher power.

> Recovery is a process of complete surrender in which we give up our reliance on externals to secure our identity.

Professional coaching

Professional health coaching: Professional coaching is a process that can address any area of health because it helps people to help themselves in a comprehensive and holistic approach. Consider the following characteristics and advantages of coaching:

Reliance on a commitment to a daily process: The power is in the process. According to Dan Goleman, emotional intelligence is more important to success than IQ (1). A process or person driven by emotional intelligence relies on consistent adherence to commitments to create results. The foundation of coaching is unconditional self-love that people provide for themselves through connection with their higher power.

1. Goleman, D. (1995). Emotional Intelligence: Why it can matter more than IQ. New York, NY: Bantam Books.

Demonstrated results: Professional coaching began with Tim Gallwey's discovery of a process of non-judgmental observations and questions that improved the results of tennis players (2). The process worked even if carried out by ski instructors coaching the tennis players. This led to the development of modern executive coaching. Since its inception, professional coaching has demonstrated that it can produce results in any area of life because it is a *holistic* life process.

Identify and prioritize health issues: The coaching process can be very effective in any area of health, but it takes time. It cannot address all areas of health simultaneously. In order to be manageable, health concerns must be identified and prioritized in each specific area and then addressed one-by-one in order of priority.

Question: What is the highest priority area you want to work on?

Helping others to help themselves: The awareness the coach brings to the client through questions helps the client know and help themselves better. If a person has a sufficient level of awareness, they can help themselves.

1. Goleman, D. (1995). Emotional Intelligence: Why it can matter more than IQ. New York, NY: Bantam Books.

2. Gallwey, W. T. (1977). *The Inner Game of Tennis.* New York, NY: Random House Trade Paperbacks.

How coaching works

- Humans have blindspots *by nature*

- Since, by definition, we cannot see blindspots, the coach has to see it and help us address it

- The coach helps the client to help themselves through awareness, personal responsibility, and proven daily disciplines

Exercise: Where do you need outside input?

Blindspots are areas of our life that we cannot see. Thus, we need the input of others to see them. If we are in denial, others see us better than we see ourselves. Author Kary Oberbrunner describes a process for working through pain in *The Deeper Path*. He took the time to "unwrap" his pain rather than avoid it. He found that dealing with his pain was a key to opening up the door to his potential. There are a number of issues listed below that contribute to blindspots.

> Blindspots are areas of our life that we cannot see. Thus, we need the input of others to see them.

Outside input

1. Ask your health coach or accountability partner if they sense you are unaware of issues affecting your health or in denial of them.

2. What can you do to address any existing health needs?

Factors for not addressing a serious health condition	Outside input needed (yes or no)
Lack of awareness	
Denial	
Addiction	
Existing enablers	

Inventory of the 7 areas of health

Because spiritual health is the only type of health that allows us to be healthy under any circumstances, it is the highest priority health area. People put themselves under enormous pressure when other areas of health become the most important. For example, most men will struggle with making work their top priority throughout their lives.

Question: What do you depend on for security?

The importance of spiritual health

Spiritual health is the only type of health that allows us to be healthy under any circumstances.

"Jesus replied: 'Love the Lord your God with all your heart and with all your soul and with all your mind.' [38]This is the first and greatest commandment.

[39]And the second is like it: 'Love your neighbor as yourself'" (Matthew 22: 37–39).

"I pray that out of his glorious riches he may strengthen you with power through his Spirit in your inner being, [17]so that Christ may dwell in your hearts through faith. And I pray that you, being rooted and established in love, [18]may have power, together with all the Lord's holy people, to grasp how wide and long and high and deep is the love of Christ, [19]and to know this love that surpasses knowledge—that you may be filled to the measure of all the fullness of God. [20]Now to him who is able to do immeasurably more than all we ask or imagine, according to his power that is at work within us, [21]to him be glory in the church and in Christ Jesus throughout all generations, for ever and ever! Amen" (Ephesians 3:16–21).

"[11]I don't say this out of need, for I have learned to be content in whatever circumstances I am. [12]I know both how to have a little, and I know how to have a lot. In any and all circumstances I have learned the secret of being content—whether well fed or hungry, whether in abundance or in need. [13]I am able to do all things through Him who strengthens me" (Philippians 4:11–13).

Scripture clarifies that our relationship with God is the most important relationship of all. He is the only One who can enable contentment in any circumstance. It is an unshakable foundation. Such a foundation is needed to prepare us for whatever comes into our lives. At some point, all of us experience tragedy and crisis.

Foundational areas of health: A self-assessment for each area of health is provided below. It was designed to illustrate the foundational nature of spiritual, relational, and emotional health. Why is spiritual health the most foundational? It is the only area of health independent of circumstances and relationship issues. History demonstrates that spiritual health has the capacity to overcome adversity even when all other areas are negative. For example, Betsy Ten Boom was observed to have consistent joy from her faith during her nine months in the concentration camp where she died.

Collier, J. (Director). (n.d.). *The Hiding Place*[Video file]. Retrieved November 6, 2017, from https://www.youtube.com/watch?v=XX0GwjXExFE

Question: What are your thoughts about the Ten Boom story?

Physical health is not foundational because a person can be physically well and yet unwell in every other area of health. Physical wellness can only supplement the other areas of health. The degree to which physical wellness helps the other areas is limited. In contrast, spiritual, relational, emotional, and mental health have much larger long-term impacts on health. Even if someone has a serious physical disability, non-physical health can enable the person to be positive, in spite of the disability. Non-physical health can overcome even the worst physical health problems whereas physical health cannot overcome problems with non-physical health.

7 types of personal health

- Spiritual health: healthy faith
- Relational health: healthy family, friends, and community
- Emotional health: emotional intelligence
- Mental health: healthy thought patterns and focus; lifelong learning

- Vocational health: healthy workplace culture and job satisfaction
- Physical health: healthy food and exercise
- Financial health: sustainable finances

Health categorization	
Area of health	**Type of health**
1. Spiritual	Foundational
2. Relational	Foundational
3. Emotional	Foundational
4. Mental	Foundational
5. Physical	Non-Foundational
6. Vocational	Non-Foundational
7. Financial	Non-Foundational

Exercise: Personal health assessment

1. Rank your health from 1–10 in each area of health, with 10 being the best on the left side of the table below.

2. Based on the score in each area, prioritize the areas in order of need on the right side of the table below from 1–7.

Health ranking	**Recovery Priority**
Spiritual	
Relational	
Emotional	

Mental	
Vocational	
Physical	
Financial	

Exercise: Evaluation of Health Priorities

1. In which areas of health are you strongest? How did you rank these areas?

2. In which areas of health are you weakest? How did you rank these areas?

A recovery approach helps us identify and acknowledge that a problem exists. We can only address problems that we are aware of. Acknowledgment that damage to our health is occurring leads to self-corrective action such as health plan implementation. Health plan implementation is a problem-solution approach free of self-judgment. Since self-judgment will inhibit recovery, it needs to be removed as we work through health problems. Therefore, health coaching specifically and intentionally removes self-judgment so that the process can work.

A recovery inventory can be performed for any of the seven areas of health. When an inventory reveals an area where damage is occurring, we acknowledge the damaging behavior and make amends. For example, if we are damaging ourselves physically through our diet and lack of exercise, we can make amends to ourselves by eating healthy food and exercising regularly.

Exercise: Stress Level Analysis

1. Stress is one of the most tangible factors we can use to monitor all the other areas of health. How can you plan to reduce your stress levels in each area of health? Use this plan to implement your stress amends. The simpler the plan, the better. If you can think of one healthy choice in each category that has an impact on the top stressor in each category, you will make progress.

	Stress Level Analysis	
Area of health	**Stress level**	**Date of next stress self-assessment**
Spiritual		
Relational		
Emotional		
Mental		
Vocational		
Physical		
Financial		

	Stress Reduction Plan	
Area of health	**Top Stressor**	**Healthy Choice**
Spiritual		
Relational		

Emotional		
Mental		
Vocational		
Physical		
Financial		

Discuss your stress reduction plan with your coach or account-ability partner and make any adjustments needed.

Exercise: Acute versus chronic pain

Question: How much pain does each of the following cause you (10 is the highest) on the scale? How long have you lived with this pain?

Condition	Pain level (1–10)	Duration
Decreased mobility		
Stress from health concerns		
Social rejection		
Financial burden (medical bills)		
Vocational burden (health-related hindrances to work)		
Spiritual burden		

Question: How much gain does each of the following cause you? How long does this gain last?

Condition	Gain level (1–10)	Duration
Exercise		
Eating healthy food		
Eating less		
Thinking less about food		
Looking and feeling better		
More mobility at work		
Peace of mind/ less brain fog		

Question: Which health gains from the table above do you connect with the most?

Question: What would you add or subtract from the list?

Question: What helps you focus on the benefits of health gains?

Exercise: Health resources for each area of health

Evaluation of time invested in each area of health			
Area of health	Self Analysis		Professional evaluation done?
	How much time invested?	Online assessment done?	
Spiritual			
Relational			
Emotional			
Mental			
Vocational			
Physical			
Financial			

1. Rate yourself from 1–10 for time invested in a health area. Ten is the best.

2. Which areas need the most attention?

3. Complete an online assessment for your top 3 areas of need. You can do additional health assessments or all of them if desired.

Health resources for each area of health

Some areas of health are difficult to measure. However, the following is a starting place for measures of each type of health:

Online Assessments	
Spiritual	http://danielplan.com/toolsandresources/healthassessment/
Relational	http://www.gottman.com/gottman-relationship-checkup/
Emotional	http://www.haygroup.com/leadershipandtalentondemand/ourproducts/item_details.aspx?itemid=58&type=1 http://www.eiconsortium.org/measures/measures.html
Mental	http://portal.mybrainfitlife.com/new/index.php/bha2/introhttps://cdn.psychologytoday.com/tests
Vocational	http://www.talentsmart.com/services/assessment-services.php
Financial	http://money.cnn.com/tools/financialhealth/

How physical health and non-physical health help each other

Exercise: Relationship of physical health to other areas of health

Positive life change tends to be the strongest and longest lasting motivation to improve and maintain health. Health improvement in the seven areas of health tends to reinforce

> Positive life change tends to be the strongest and longest lasting motivation to improve and maintain health.

each other and synergize to create both momentum and endurance.

1. List your top reason for how better physical health will help each of the other main areas of health in the table below. For example, reduced stress could be a reason in several or all categories.

How physical health helps non-physical health	
Area of health	**How does physical health help non-physical health?**
Spiritual	
Relational	
Emotional	
Mental	
Vocational	
Financial	

2. List your top reason why each area of non-physical health below helps your physical health.

How non-physical health helps physical health	
Area of health	**How is physical health helped by non-physical health?**
Spiritual	
Relational	
Emotional	

Mental	
Vocational	
Financial	

3. Share your answers. What reasons stand out?

Community aspect of recovery

Root Causes: In order to address the root causes of health problems, participation in an ongoing identity-based recovery program is a foundational step. Without an ongoing recovery program, the chances of regaining weight and health relapses are high. Identity healing is the foundation for every type of health issue.

Holistic recovery provides the energy we need to improve our health. Without sufficient levels of foundational health, we won't have the energy or the clarity to go the extra mile in the non-foundational areas (physical, vocational, and financial). Increasing capacity means uncovering all the defects that impact our spiritual, relational, emotional, and mental health one at a time. If we are completely honest with ourselves and our recovery community about uncovering our hurts, habits, and hangups, the recovery process will help us convert the pain into potential.

Celebrate Recovery (CR) is recommended as a recovery community for the following reasons:

- *Identity-based:* CR programs are applicable to any area of recovery because identity issues are at the center of any non-physical health problem.

- *Consistency:* The CR recovery model has been worked out over the course of more than 25 years. All CR programs have the same structure.

- *Community-based:* Small groups provide a combination of support, confidentiality, and accountability. It is a safe environment.

- *Availability:* Recovery issues can occur anywhere, especially when traveling. You can attend a meeting in any major city when traveling.

Participants may choose an alternative identity-based program, but it should meet the above criteria.

Exercise: Selection of a recovery community

John Bradshaw concludes that the vast majority of Americans struggle with addiction, whether it is recognized as addiction or not (1). Everyone needs a support system and a recovery community because everyone has some area of health that needs attention. A good example is Robert Lewis' 33 series men's ministry (2). It is community- and recovery-oriented, even though it is not officially labeled as a recovery group. Functionally, it is a recovery group.

1. Bradshaw, J. (2012). The role of shame in addiction. The Meadows. Retrieved from https://www.themeadows.com/blog/item/152-the-role-of-shame-in-addiction

2. Authentic Manhood. (n.d.). 33: The series. Retrieved from https://www.authenticmanhood.com

Question: What are your thoughts on attending a group that helps strengthen identity? Attendance may help you overcome a non-traditional addiction that is taking up too much time and energy (work, food, sports, entertainment).

Review groups you are currently involved in. Do they identify areas of health that need to be addressed and provide a path toward recovery? Fill in the table below:

Group	Identification of needs	Provision of a recovery process
1.		
2.		
3.		

If you do not have a recovery community, review available options and try one out within the next week.

Group Options	Time	Place
1. Celebrate Recovery		
2. Community group		

3. Church group		
4. _______		

If attending for the first time, how did your group go?

____

____

____

____

____

____

Helping others helps us

Question: What is your favorite way to help others?

Question: What benefits do you notice when you volunteer?

Exercise: How to begin the process of helping someone in need

Think through people you already know. Who is struggling with their physical health?

Could you ask:

- About their health status?
- Are they open to being helped with wellness issues?

- Would they consider reading material on wellness or type 2 diabetes?

What can you do to help them?

- If they express openness to wellness improvement, invite them into a mentoring process.
- Begin taking them through these exercises and fine-tune the process according to the specific situation.

13

HOW DOES HEALTH COACHING HELP?

Why is non-physical health more important than physical health?

COACHING INVOLVES THE whole person. Each person has 7 different components that make up their life. Most of these are non-physical: spiritual, emotional, mental, relational. Thus, there are four areas of non-physical health and one area of physical health. Good non-physical health always improves whatever our current physical state is.

The internally-based areas of non-physical health form an even more important subcategory. Emotional, mental, and spiritual health can remain stable and healthy in spite of external circumstances by self-management of our thoughts. Relational health can be included in this category in terms of our relationship with ourselves. If our relationship with ourselves is healthy, it always improves our relationships with others and vice versa. Coaching places particular emphasis on improving this relationship with ourselves.

How to build a healthy brain

The brain is the most important organ we can use to help ourselves. Dr. Daniel Amen is a brain health expert who pioneered the use of SPECT scans to analyze the brain and prescribe treatments. His basic brain health strategy includes exercise, a healthy breakfast, effective stress management, and more than 6 hours of sleep. Exercise is important because it increases blood flow to the brain. Insufficient sleep decreases cognitive function.

The Daniel Plan highlights common symptoms of stress and how to address them. The following steps are suggested for stress management:

- Pray on a regular basis by substituting prayer for worry. This substitution can turn something negative into something positive

- Delegate and minimize overscheduling

- Listen to soothing music

- Use calming scented materials such as lavender

- Use calming supplements

- Laugh more

- Challenge automatic negative thoughts (ANTs) and replace them with truthful thoughts. ANTs include:
  - overgeneralizations such as always and never
  - an over-reliance on feelings without determining the validity of the thoughts behind the feelings

- o   forecasting the future
- o   blaming
- o   denial
- o   focusing on the negative
- Successful strategies for countering negative thoughts include:
  - o   generating a gratitude list which becomes the focus of the first seven minutes of the day
  - o   stop triggers from becoming a negative perception
  - o   view failure as growth
  - o   SMART goals (Specific, Measurable, Aligned, Realistic, Time-bound)

Priorities are another area where stress can be addressed. Multi-tasking creates stress by dividing our attention between too many priorities. In contrast, focusing on the top priority step-by-step decreases stress because this strategy provides a valid sense of progress toward meaningful goals. According to John Maxwell, success in any area includes relationship building, equipping/training people, positive attitude, and leadership (1). Prioritizing these areas in projects, meetings, and proposals can move us in the right direction.

John Maxwell designs his schedule according to his priorities by matching his most productive time of the day with his highest priorities. For 35 years, he has kept mornings free for his strengths; he does lower priorities at night, tasks that don't require a fresh mind. He also employs his staff to help him manage meeting priorities and screen requests.

1.   Maxwell, J. C. (2011). *How to be a Real success.* Duluth, GA: The John Maxwell Company.

What is coaching?

Christian Simpson is the lead faculty member for the John Maxwell Team coaching program, a leadership organization that trains people to speak, coach, and lead. He explains the underlying basis of coaching, individual coaching skills, and the coaching process. You can review options for training at www.johnmaxwellgroup.com.

Coaching utilizes emotional intelligence and the enormous resources of the subconscious mind to help people express more of their potential. According to Bruce Lipton, the subconscious mind has a processing capacity of 4 billion bits per second compared to 2000 bits per second in the conscious mind (1). The beliefs residing in the unconscious mind control our lives. Subconscious beliefs about ourselves are the ultimate cause of our behaviors. Until these beliefs are made conscious and forged in a positive direction through personal growth, our behavior patterns will not change. Coaching is perhaps the only known process that can change subconscious beliefs.

> Subconscious beliefs about ourselves are the ultimate cause of our behaviors.

Conscious inputs, in combination with follow-up actions, can eventually become new subconscious beliefs. This process involves the transformation from unconscious incompetence to unconscious competence. This transformation is a difficult process that requires a positive focus on potential instead of existing results and circumstances. Coaching helps people to help transform themselves by engaging them in a daily process of personal growth that moves them toward their potential through emotional intelligence. Coaching places far greater emphasis on emotional intelligence (EQ) than IQ because EQ is a far greater determinant of success and quality of life.

1. Bruce Lipton. (n.d.). What would your life be like if you learned that you are more powerful than you have ever been taught?. Mountain of Love Productions. Retrieved from https://www.brucelipton.com/

The coaching process itself is based on questions with the following characteristics:

- curiosity-based
- open-ended
- non-judgmental

As coaching questions are asked, the conscious mind engages the question and searches the subconscious mind for the answer. As this process is repeated and reinforced through daily personal growth and follow-up action, new subconscious beliefs are eventually realized.

The ongoing need for coaching

According to TalentSmart, emotional intelligence (EQ) skills are more important to job performance than any other skill set because relationships are how work gets done. In others words, leaders and managers get work done through people. Middle managers had the highest EQ scores. Above middle management, there's a steep downward trend in EQ. CEOs on average have the lowest EQ scores in the workplace (1).

Talentsmart also discovered year-to-year trends in emotional intelligence varied with the economy. Emotional intelligence dipped significantly during the Great Recession 2008–2009 (1). This may help explain the drop in EQ above middle management. The higher pressure there tends to push emotional intelligence to a lower priority. However, this is precisely the opportunity for emotional intelligence skills to shine the brightest.

According to TalentSmart, the following are some best practices that are helpful in self-management and emotional intelligence:

- Take control of yourself talk: Self-talk thoughts are the most influential thoughts because our internal voices affect our perceptions of our environments.

- Thoughts are primary regulator of emotional flow: Self-talk damages your ability to self-manage any time it becomes negative. Turning negative self-talk into positive self-talk can increase the ability to self-manage. For example, change the statements "I always" or "I never" into "I sometimes." Replace judgmental statements like "I'm an idiot" with factual ones like "I made a mistake." Focus thoughts on your actions and not the actions of others.

- Seek advice from a trustworthy person who is not personally affected by your situation. They can provide more objective feedback.

- Become a learner from every person you encounter: Approaching people you encounter as though they have something valuable to teach you is the best way to remain flexible, open-minded, and less stressed.

- Include mental recharge in your schedule: This activity is as important to your brain as healthy food is to your body. Energy management is key to self-management.

1. Bradberry, T., & Greaves, J. (2009). Emotional intelligence 2.0. San Diego, CA: TalentSmart.

Can coaching change lifelong eating habits?

> Professional coaching is a sustainable means of behavior change because it helps people to help themselves.

Professional coaching is a sustainable means of behavior change because it helps people to help themselves. By changing limiting beliefs in the subconscious mind, it does more to move a person closer to their potential than conventional human developmental processes. As limiting beliefs are replaced by beliefs in personal potential, capacity increases in all areas of health (1).

Coaching is useful for helping people change unhealthy eating behaviors and low activity levels. Changing lifelong eating habits is notoriously difficult. There are deeply held beliefs lying below conscious awareness that reinforce unhealthy eating habits. Coaching can expose these beliefs and facilitate their replacement by beliefs that support long-term health.

Michael F. Roizen, MD, is the Chief Wellness Officer at Cleveland Clinic. He routinely takes patients at the Cleveland Clinic Wellness Institute who are in the midst of struggling with tobacco, heart, diabetic, or arthritic problems and coaches them with simple (but persistent) lifestyle changes to help them live, feel, and look years younger. He enjoys helping them get off meds and teaches the role of food and other simple steps in reversing disease processes. Cleveland Clinic Wellness Institute aims to elevate preventive care and wellness as a core brand and a core value that they teach their patients and employees.

Dr. Roizen cited the following preventative healthcare processes to facilitate successful reversal of diet-driven disease:

- Accountability partner or health coach
- Successful introductions of a new health habit
- Successful introductions of a second health habit
- Stress management
- Mediterranean diet

According to Dr. Roizen, "The trick is infusing diet knowledge into the patient" repeatedly (2). Health coaching is the key to successful change. Test results typically result in a temporary change followed by a reversion back to previous behaviors. Dr. Roizen has a daily accountability program with the people he coaches.

1. The John Maxwell Team. (n.d.). The John Maxwell Team Vision. Retrieved from www.johnmaxwellgroup.com

2. How healthcare impacts community sustainability [Interview by T. Schierer]. (2016, December 28). Interview with Dr. Mike Roizen at the Cleveland Clinic

Why are eating habits so hard to change?

Awareness of the importance of emotional intelligence (EQ) has grown since the 1990s after the publication of *Emotional Intelligence* by Dan Goleman. EQ is a far greater determinant of performance than IQ. One of the main reasons for this is that most of the brain's activity occurs in the subconscious part of the mind. Emotional memory houses subconscious memories, values, and belief systems that drive our behavior (1).

Decisions to eat unhealthy food are driven by subconscious emotional memory far more than cognitive decisions. Once healthy beliefs replace unhealthy beliefs in the subconscious mind, the subconscious mind will drive new behaviors. Professional coaching is the most effective process known for converting unhealthy subconscious beliefs to healthy subconscious beliefs (1).

1. The John Maxwell Team. (n.d.). The John Maxwell Team Vision. Retrieved from www.johnmaxwellgroup.com

Can cravings change within a week?

Most people struggle with craving unhealthy foods at some level. These cravings can be reduced from a daily occurrence to a weekly or monthly occurrence. Cravings are never completely eliminated, but they can be increasingly converted to healthy cravings. For example, cravings for desserts can be changed to craving healthy, whole food smoothies. Cravings can change so dramatically that comfort foods become repulsive to the body and mind.

> People notice a major shift in cravings within 4–10 days.

The craving conversion process includes both coaching and dietary facilitators. Healthy fat, fiber, and water consumption combine to help people feel full and satisfied. Fibers such as glucomannan absorb several times their weight in water. As a result, people feel full without over-consuming calories. This combination controls cravings very well. People notice a major shift in cravings within 4 days. (1)

1. Hyman, M. (n.d.). 10 day detox diet starter kit. Retrieved from http://www.10daydetoxcookbook. com/?a_aid=54ef3e65242a0&a_ bid=944fd4dd&chan=code4

How a healthy fat diet makes it easier to change eating habits (1)

Why we are "always hungry" on a high-carb diet

- Consumption of simple carbohydrates leads to the production of insulin

- Insulin stimulates fat cells to hoard glucose from the blood, leaving too few calories for the rest of the body

- The brain senses low blood sugar and thinks that we're hungry because all the calories are hidden inside the fat cells

How to program our brain and body to sense that we are not starving (2)

- High healthy fat diets decrease insulin production

- Fat cells are no longer stimulated to hoard calories by insulin spikes

- Fat cells in non-hoarding mode can now begin to release calories back into the body, and the brain no longer thinks we are calorie-deprived

- Hunger lessens

Summary of how a healthy fat diet helps reverse diabetes

- High healthy fat / low-carb diets result in less insulin production

- The reduction of insulin spikes brings insulin release back into balance

- Balanced levels of insulin prevent the pancreas from being overworked and prevent our body from becoming more insulin-resistant

1. Ludwig, D. (2016). Always hungry: Conquer cravings, retrain your fat cells, and lose weight permanently. New York, NY: Grand Central Publishing.

2. Hyman, M. (n.d.). How to rewire your brain to end food cravings. Dr. Hyman. Retrieved from http://drhyman.com/blog/2012/03/01/how-to-rewire-your-brain-to-end-food-cravings/

PART 3

HOW TO BUILD STRONGER COMMUNITIES THROUGH WELLNESS OUTREACH

14

50/25: HOW TO BUILD STRONGER COMMUNITIES THROUGH WELLNESS

Will 40 years of high-carb, low-fat frustration transform into a wellness movement?

ACCORDING TO A study by Rocca et al., declines in heart disease and stroke mortality rates are conventionally attributed to reductions in cigarette smoking, recognition and treatment of hypertension and diabetes, effective medications to improve serum lipid levels and to reduce clot formation, and general lifestyle improvements (1). Modern medical treatments are scientifically advanced and have lengthened lives that would have been cut short in previous generations.

Most people want to be healthy, but many have been frustrated by low-fat, high-carb diets of the last 40 or more years. The low-fat craze is subsiding, but the weight loss frustration and the chronic disease it produced may generate a massive wellness movement in the opposite direction of its original intent. If a wellness movement arises from low-fat, high-carb, it will be because it generated most of the chronic diseases plaguing America. As mentioned here and by many other authors, the low-fat craze was a main contributor to our epidemics of diabetes, obesity, heart disease, and Alzheimer's. Government food pyramids and the intentional suppression of alternative views by academics and federal oversight committees allowed the low-fat craze to take hold (2). Most citizens, doctors, and scientists remained in the dark for 40–60 years.

This length of time then allowed massive epidemics of diet-driven chronic disease to be generated. 50% of Americans are prediabetic or diabetic (3) because the Standard American Diet (SAD) generates type 2 diabetes. Doctors began to doubt the food pyramids when too many of their patients were getting sick following the food pyramid. In response to the mounting evidence against high-carb, low-fat, the government food nutrition recommendations changed in 2015 to declare dietary cholesterol as an issue no longer of concern (4). As this information becomes more widely known, light bulbs are appearing over the heads of an increasing number of citizens. This information brings to the surface the questions that have been beneath the surface for many years:

- Why is America so fat and so sick?
- Why do so many people struggle to keep weight off?
- Why do people lose weight by eating fat?
- Why is the rest of the world getting fat and sick on American fast food?

These questions have readied people to receive and understand the new healthy fat studies. People know it's true because the evidence is all around us. The level of frustration generated by 70 years of chronic disease can be a strong impetus for a wellness movement that achieves high levels of momentum. Such a movement may even be likely, given that medium- to high-fat, *non-deprivation* diets are one of the best answers to low-fat, high-carb deprivation diets. People trying to lose weight on low-fat, high-carb diets wanted wellness but were literally defeating themselves. A high-fat wellness movement will not be self-defeating because it works with the natural design of our metabolism.

> The level of frustration generated by 70 years of chronic disease can be a strong impetus for a wellness movement that achieves high levels of momentum.

High-fat diets are not a cure-all for everyone (5), but they will probably work well for most people. The best diet is always the one individualized to a person's genetic makeup, culture, and lifestyle. No diet can overcome poor non-physical health. Stress hormones stimulated by insufficient levels of stress management can be such a powerful negative force that it can negate the effects of a healthy physical lifestyle. Poor non-physical health can arise from a variety of situations:

- Divorce
- Mental illness
- High work stress
- Poor job fit

1. Rocca, W. A., et al. (2011). Trends in the incidence and prevalence of Alzheimer's disease, dementia, and cognitive impairment in the United States, Alzheimer's & Dementia, 7(1), 80-93. doi:10.1016/j.jalz.2010.11.002

2. Teicholz, N. (2014). The big fat surprise: Why butter, meat and cheese belong in a healthy diet. New York, NY: Simon & Schuster Paperbacks.

3. Menke, A., et al. (2015). Prevalence of and trends in diabetes among adults in the United States, 1988-2012. European Journal of Public Health, 21, 484-490.

4. USA, USDA. (2015). Dietary Guidelines 2015-2020. Retrieved from https://health.gov/dietaryguidelines/2015/guidelines/executive-summary

5. Sears, B. (2005). The anti-inflammation zone: Reversing the silent epidemic that's destroying our health (The zone). New York, NY: HarperCollins Publishers Inc.

What factors create a self-sustaining wellness movement?

For people who have good non-physical health, a huge boost of momentum will be gained as they begin to implement this new wave of information on healthy fat, Mediterranean-style diets, and functional medicine diets. They will notice massive differences in cravings, energy, mental alertness, attitude, and of course a thinner, leaner body that doesn't require calorie counting. This kind of life change creates advocates of change on a community scale. A change this massive creates leaders who believe in the movement and want to make a difference. A number of different elements can and will likely come together to create a self-sustaining wellness movement with high levels of momentum:

- **Wellness movement initiator:** The experience of high levels of personal change will be the main movement driver. This will be helped by the desire to lose weight in a way, that works with our metabolism instead of against it.

- **Wellness momentum maintainer:** The desire to stay at a high level of health will be a self-sustaining, built-in mechanism to maintain the momentum of community wellness.

- **Connection driver:** The strength of wellness as a generator of common ground will facilitate the desire to connect with others in the movement and facilitate the ease of those connections.

- **Food infrastructure change driver:** Widespread knowledge of the chronic disease effects of low-fat, high-carb will be a powerful driver of consumer choices away from high-sugar, processed foods toward delicious, healthy functional medicine style choices. Consumer demand can change what the food industry produces.

- **Community change driver:** The high levels of momentum and common ground generated by wellness can spill over into other areas of community sustainability where there is less agreement and drive positive change in areas such as workplace engagement and soil and water conservation.

This powerful combination of momentum factors will be strong enough to initiate change in the American food industry. When consumers begin purchasing mostly or only healthy food and stop purchasing unhealthy food, food manufacturers and restaurants will change in order to stay in business. Soft drink manufacturers have responded to the steady decline in soda sales by bringing healthier, unsweetened drinks to the market. Consumers can drive change in our food infrastructure with their purchasing power. Because at least 50% of Americans are likely to be ready to end the cycle of feeling sick and fat, there is sufficient reason to believe that a self-sustaining wellness movement will become a reality. In the coming decades, we will witness the reduction, disappearance, or transformation of:

- Shelves of processed foods at grocery stores
- Walls of sweetened drinks at convenience stores
- Ice cream and dessert stores
- Traditional fast food
- Chronic disease: T2D, heart disease, cancer, Alzheimer's

After 60 years of misinformation and visible results of that misinformation, it is not likely that people will continue to believe advertising for fast food, beverage, and dessert industries. Even though the established food industry is large and powerful, they are dependent on consumer choice. They will be forced to change once consumers no longer buy high-carb, low-fat or highly processed products.

The main inhibitor of the wellness movement will be the slow nature of behavior change. Cravings and habits can take many years to overcome. Therefore, people will continue buying too many sweets and high-carb foods which generate cravings. In addition, advertising of unhealthy food and beverage choices will remain prominent as long as they are profitable. People do not change rapidly; they must fail repeatedly over several years before cravings and eating behaviors change long-term. The majority of people who have not yet gained control of their cravings will succumb to the high availability of unhealthy food and drink. But slowly, change will come. Each year, the desire for personal change will grow stronger until it takes hold. Ultimately, most people will adopt long-term change if they realize that better, non-deprivation diets exist.

Why will it be different this time? What will keep people from regaining the weight that they lost? This time, weight loss will be based on non-deprivation diets. People will feel full, satisfied, and healthy as they lose weight, not sick and deprived. This is the nature of change on a healthy fat diet. The weight comes off naturally. It gives long-term strugglers a starting point without needing to bring excess exercise into the picture. Diet and exercise are no longer insurmountable barriers for overweight and obese individuals who have struggled with their weight for decades.

Wellness creates common ground

Stanford University published a model for community service collaboration called Collective Impact. It is based on the principle of finding common ground with individual or organizational collaborators. The principle of finding common ground can be the starting point for collaboration on even difficult problems. The problems people have in common are greater than the problems that separate them. Chronic disease is perhaps the largest common problem.

Wellness is a practical means of averting broader community crises. Perhaps for the first time in history, ordinary citizens have the tools to make a difference in the

> The economic burden of chronic disease consumes over 80% of American health care costs.

broader economy. Since the economic burden of chronic disease consumes over 80% of American health care costs (1), large-scale public health can positively impact the national economy. Wellness helps all parts of the community through greater productivity and lower costs. Therefore, wellness is a viable means of community sustainability. A strategy for achieving community sustainability through wellness, workplace engagement, soil and water conservation, and leadership development is provided in the following section.

1. Aldridge, M. D., & Kelley, A. S. (2015). The myth regarding the high cost of end-of-life care. American Journal of Public Health, 105(12), 2411-2415. doi:10.2105/AJPH.2015.302889

How to build stronger communities through wellness

As discussed, the motivational rationale for a wellness movement is based on the long-term frustration of entire nations struggling to keep weight off. Many people are genuinely frustrated with calorie counting, regaining weight, and the psychological burden of deprivation diets. If a non-deprivation alternative is what people need, what would hold them back from relieving themselves of the frustration of deprivation diets? Therefore, the motivational rationale has a solid, long-term basis. The structural framework facilitating the wellness movement is based on making a difference at both the individual and organizational levels. Wellness is a natural bridge builder in building communities and can function at both of these levels. A basic strategy for achieving long-term community sustainability based on wellness is outlined below:

50/25 strategy for community building through wellness

Overall goals
50 At least 50% of the US population is involved in targeted, ongoing volunteerism.
25 At least 25% of the US population is involved in holistic personal wellness programs that increase personal sustainability and capacity.

What is the foundation of community sustainability?

- **Wellness:** Holistic preventative healthcare ultimately impacts every type of sustainability more than any other approach

- **Community:** Use of talents, interests, skills, personality, and experiences to impact the community positively. Everyone has something to contribute (Warren, R. 2012).
  - Warren, R. (2012). The Purpose Driven Life. Grand Rapids, MI: Zondervan.

What are the sustainability priorities needed for a viable sustainability movement?

1. Personal health

2. Community health

3. Vocational health

4. Environmental health

Priority sustainability needs	
Area of need	**Scope of need**
Personal health	69% of US population over-weight (1)
	84% of healthcare costs are preventable (2)
	50% with one or more chronic diseases (3)
	Socially acceptable addiction is close to 100% in the U.S. (food, entertainment, sports)
Community health	58% of the federal budget is spent on healthcare and welfare; most programs are dependency-based (4)
Vocational health	71% disengaged at the workplace (5)
Environmental health	50% of Midwest topsoil eroded (6)
	Africa will have the most people and the least water by 2100 (7)
	Amazon rainforest may hit critical deforestation threshold within 20 years (8)

1. National Institute of Diabetes and Digestive and Kidney Diseases. (2012). Overweight & obesity statistics. Retrieved from https://www.niddk.nih.gov/health-information/health-statistics/Pages/overweight-obesity-statistics.aspx

2. *Moses H 3rd, Matheson DH, Dorsey ER, George BP, Sadoff D, Yoshimura S JAMA. 2013 Nov 13; 310(18):1947-63.* doi: 10.1001/jama.2013.281425.

3. Menke, A., et al. (2015). Prevalence of and trends in diabetes among adults in the United States. JAMA, 314(10), 1021-1029. doi:10.1001/jama.2015.10029

4. Lundeen, A. (2014, April). Where do your federal tax dollars go?. Tax Foundation. Retrieved from https://taxfoundation.org/where-do-your-tax-dollars-go/

5. Business Journal. (2002, April). The high cost of disengaged employees. Business Journal. Retrieved from http://www.gallup.com/businessjournal/247/the-high-cost-of-disengaged-employees.aspx

6. Arsenault, C. (n.d.). Only 60 years of farming left if soil degradation continues. Scientific American. Retrieved from https://www.scientificamerican.com/article/only-60-years-of-farming-left-if-soil-degradation-continues/

7. Engelman, R. (2016). Six billion in Africa. Scientific American, 314(2), 56-63. doi:10.1038/scientificamerican0216-56

8. Soares-Filho, B. S., et al. (2006) Modelling conservation in the Amazon basin. Nature, 440(7083), 520-523.

Top 4 priority sustainability target areas	
Area of need	**Sustainability target areas**
Personal health	Preventative healthcare
Community health	Leadership-based social programs
Vocational health	Leadership culture building and workplace engagement
Environmental health	Soil and water conservation

Priority sustainability networks	
Area of need	**Type of sustainability networks**
Personal health	Preventative healthcare networks
Community health	**Community networks:** NGO, GOV, BIZ **Sector networks:** NGO, GOV, BIZ **Influence networks:** education, government, media, ministry, business, arts/entertainment, family

Vocational health	Leadership and coaching networks
Environmental health	Soil and water sustainability networks

NGO: non-governmental organization
GOV: government organization
BIZ: business sector

Networking Process

Purpose: to network organizations that through various local and national combinations can enable staff in all 7 areas of health according to their organizational expertise.

Who can benefit from the 50/25 sustainability network?

People and organizations who can help people in any of the 7 areas of health according to their personal or organizational expertise. The 7 areas of health include: relational, emotional, mental, spiritual, physical, financial, and vocational health.

- Local lead agencies:
  1. Prioritize areas of health in greatest need according to local agency data.
  2. Prioritize the local agencies that have the highest impact in the areas of greatest need.

- Regional and national organizations:
  1. Partner with local organizations to support projects within priority sustainability areas.

2. Implement larger projects requiring the resources of a large organization or network of larger organizations according to sustainability priorities.

How does the 50/25 sustainability network function?

A 50/25 sustainability network functions through sustainability priorities, repetition, common networking method, and scalability.

Sustainability priorities: 50/25 goals require a national network of lead agencies in the 7 areas of health who cooperate because they are aware of sustainability priorities and the potential sustainability tipping points. Sustainability priorities enable cooperation through a common agenda.

- 50% targeted volunteerism: The U.S. has over 1 million non-profits, including hundreds in priority sustainability areas; a doubling of the current volunteer rate is achievable. People can and will choose to volunteer when they clearly see:
  - Benefits of volunteering to their own lives: Helping others helps us.
  - Volunteering has a vital role in national and local sustainability for current and future generations.
- 25% involvement in holistic wellness is possible when the variety of available programs is considered.
  - Holistic wellness programs can function as recovery programs. The percent of the population who care about their health enough to be physically active is about 60%. Currently active individuals may be open to taking the additional step toward

including non-physical areas of health in their personal care. If people see non-physical areas of health as essential to their wellness, they will become open to participation in holistic recovery.

- o There are a wide variety of other recovery-based programs that can help achieve holistic personal sustainability:

  - community groups

  - wellness groups

  - men's groups

  - women's groups

  - church groups

  - mindfulness groups

  - mentoring groups

  - recovery groups

  - sports groups

Repetition: A network of agencies can help ensure sufficient repetition for behavior change. People generally take a single improvement step or a few steps from any single wellness program, even though the program may offer more. People adopt healthy habits in response to *repetitive messages from a wide variety of sources*. When diverse organizations reinforce the same message, people tend to believe those messages. A network that is too small won't provide sufficient repetition from a wide enough variety of sources to initiate behavior change. A network of organizations

> People adopt healthy habits in response to *repetitive messages from a wide variety of sources.*

helps people and communities change more than any one organization.

Common networking method: Stanford's Collective Impact model in combination with the Intentional Living model developed by the John Maxwell Company. Collective Impact provides the guidelines for organizational collaboration, and Intentional Living provides a model for making a daily difference in the lives of those in our community.

Collective Impact summary

- Common agenda: Sustainability targets
- Shared measurement systems: Sustainability metrics
- Mutually reinforcing activities: Sustainability networks
- Continuous communication: Sustainability networks
- Backbone support organizations: Sustainability networks
- Effective decision-making: Sustainability priorities

Intentional Living summary

- People making a difference: Everyone has interests, talents, resources, and experiences in sustainability priority areas.
- Doing something that makes a difference: Everyone can make a difference in and for the community in sustainability priority areas.
- With people who make a difference: Community sustainability is accomplished *together* through a network of organizations and communities.

- At a time that makes a difference: Communities may begin to experience the consequences of sustainability tipping points within the next 30 years.

Scalability: Individuals and organizations can benefit from sustainability priorities, strategies, and networks. The number and type of individuals and organizations can expand indefinitely because sustainability priorities are based on fundamental human and environmental needs.

Common approach: The 50/25 strategy is the common approach. It addresses the root cause of all sustainability issues: unsustainable human behavior. The more people are involved in making a positive difference in their community according to sustainability priorities, the more sustainable it will become.

> The more people are involved in making a positive difference in their community according to sustainability priorities, the more sustainable it will become.

Prioritization: Goals that are not prioritized according to sustainability needs will not likely create sufficient levels of sustainability.

Flexibility: Within the overall sustainability priorities, individuals, groups, and communities have wide flexibility in choosing where they make a sustainability impact. 50/25 sustainability priorities can fit into any collaborating organization's existing mission and vision because the priorities listed above are based on fundamental human and environmental needs.

Adaptability: As sustainability metrics provide increasing clarity, some sustainability priorities may require increased emphasis and other areas may require decreased emphasis. For example, it is possible that large numbers of people may engage in wellness behaviors that preclude the need for excessive healthcare expenditures. These resources could then be directed towards the new number one sustainability priority.

4 Basic subgoals

- *Establish a national network of organizations* that agree on data-based sustainability priorities.

- *Target volunteer activities* of organizations in the network according to sustainability priorities.

- *Increase volunteerism level to at least 50%* in sustainability priority areas and generate a system for creating *ongoing* volunteerism.

- Increase participation in holistic wellness (physical and non-physical health) groups to 25% through sustainability priorities.

According to John Maxwell, leadership is about consistently adding value to others. This is why anyone can improve their leadership skills. People who don't consider themselves leaders can actually become skilled in leadership by becoming skilled in helping others. Helping others gives us influence with them. Influence, in turn, is leadership. Intentionally adding value to others according to prioritized processes and plans maximizes impact. Influence increases personal capacity because there is a relationship between finding your purpose and finding your energy. Increased personal capacity, in turn, increases organizational capacity. Increased organizational capacity, in turn, increases community sustainability.

How NGO's and businesses can contribute to building sustainable communities through wellness

How nonprofits can channel investment in a sustainable direction

One of the advantages of the United States is its integrated social sectors of government, business, and NGOs. It does this better than any other nation according to non-profit experts (1). These different sectors can work together to create financial sustainability by promoting the right kind of investment. Often momentum has to build in communities before the government sector is ready to participate. Volunteerism is essential to community health because of the impact it has on relationships between people and organizations. It also has an impact on people because it helps people get their focus off their problems and onto problem-solving. In this way, volunteerism increases personal capacity.

Volunteerism is one of the few activities that transcends political and belief systems. In a world of polarized beliefs that stops elected leaders from working together to solve problems, volunteerism is perhaps not only the best solution but the only practical solution to circumvent political deadlock.

> Volunteerism is one of the few activities that transcends politics and belief systems.

When people from opposite viewpoints volunteer together, it can break down barriers. This is because volunteerism, by nature, changes the focus from obstacles to what people have in common. Humans, by nature, have much in common, even regarding beliefs. For example, many people agree on the characteristics of a healthy personal identity, no matter what their religious beliefs. Specifically, people agree that people can have a secure personal identity apart from what happens to them.

1. Hopkins, B. (2017). *Starting and Managing a Non-profit organization*(7th ed.). Hoboken, NJ: John Wiley and Sons.

Are bankers wellness professionals?

Almost everyone is a health professional or is in direct contact with one because there are seven different areas of health:

- Mental Health: counselors, psychologists, psychiatrists, non-profit organizations, human service organizations, mentors, other mental health professionals

- Spiritual health: pastors, priests, lay leaders, spiritual leaders

- Emotional: counselors, recovery organizations, emotional intelligence professionals and organizations

- Relational health: counselors, recovery organizations, social organizations

- Physical health: doctors, nurses, exercise professionals, health coaches, wellness professionals, chiropractors, nutritionists

- Financial health: bankers, investors, wealth managers, financial advisors, and other financial professionals

- Vocational health: human resource directors, human capital professionals, workplace culture professionals, trainers

Many of the professionals listed above would not consider themselves health workers. Could awareness of their role as a health worker create a common cause that would direct and streamline communities towards wellness? For example, if bankers thought of themselves more as financial health workers, would it increase their impact, effectiveness, and innovation in the community? Could it stimulate more connection and collaboration with other professions in different areas of health to create diverse, problem-solving teams? Diverse teams are more likely to solve future, unforeseen challenges.

How doctors are turning good health into good biz

Dr. Mark Hyman has interviewed many different medical professionals, mainly doctors, who have turned good health into good business (1). Good health and good business are a good combination. In fact, profitable business is one of the fastest ways to create change in a capitalist democracy such as the United States.

Too much of the business sector has traditionally promoted poor physical and environmental health. The opposite can be the case: use profit to create health and environmental conservation. Without the cooperation of business, personal and environmental health will remain at risk.

We enjoy great freedoms in the U.S. However, if profit is not used to promote personal and environmental health, it will endanger our freedom. As Dr. David Ludwig of Harvard Medical School explained, widespread poor health is our most serious national security issue (2). Poor health is more likely to result in a sustainability crisis than other potential causes because of the scale of its impact.

According to Dr. David Ludwig of Harvard Medical School, widespread poor health is our most serious national security issue.

Mark Hyman and his colleagues are both successful doctors and successful business owners. Because at least half of America's population is at risk for poor health or a health crisis, there is room for an army of doctors and health professionals to create businesses that promote good health. A diversity of such businesses can be one of the anchors of a stable economy at the local level and the national level. Indeed, holistic personal health is not only the basis of personal sustainability but also the basis of financial sustainability.

1. The Fat Summit 2. (n.d.). Discover what the latest research says about eating fat!. Retrieved from http:// fatsummit.com/fat1/

2. Ludwig, D. (2016). Always hungry: Conquer cravings, retrain your fat cells, and lose weight permanently. New York, NY: Grand Central Publishing.

Pharma can create their future

Dr. Hyman has explained the importance of supplements. If we lived in the world where fresh produce was delivered locally, the soil was undegraded; there were no GMOs, no pesticides, no herbicides, and many other factors, we would not need supplements. Thus, everyone can benefit from nutritional supplements. The need is large.

The pharmaceutical industry has vast resources to create its own future. The current paradigm in healthcare has emphasized treatment over prevention. That model has not worked well for personal or community sustainability. The pharmaceutical industry spends vast sums of money on research and development and clinical trials. The clinical phase for some drugs can cost a billion dollars (1). There are obvious savings to pharma by switching to a model of prevention. Non-regulated nutritional supplements can potentially help people much more than a drug to treat disease and also avoid the vast sums spent on clinical trials. There may be as many paths to profit for the pharmaceutical industry in the health and wellness industry as in the treatment industry. As with the oil industry, pharma would do well to take their vast resources to create a future in accordance with sustainability instead of relying on an unsustainable product stream.

1. Feyman, Y. (2014). Shocking secrets of FDA clinical trials revealed. Forbes. Retrieved from http://www.forbes.com/sites/theapothecary/2014/01/24/shocking-secrets-of-fda-clinical-trials-revealed/#561164bb2279

Healthier workplaces help build healthier communities

WELCOA has been a leading organization in workplace wellness for over 20 years. Their model for workplace wellness is called the 7 Benchmarks. This model has helped hundreds of organizations to establish results-oriented workplace wellness programs. A results-oriented program gathers baseline data on which the program is built. Without the foundational wellness data, programs are usually unsuccessful. Only 7% of workplace wellness programs are considered results-oriented: a program that gathers baseline metrics on employee health and wellness interests.

Initial surveys of employee wellness interests form the foundation to start the workplace wellness program. As the program progresses, health metrics gauge progress. Another key tenet of the 7 benchmarks is establishing support from senior organizational leadership. This turns out to be one of the most critical factors in determining success. Results-oriented workplace wellness programs typically yield a 3:1 one return. Some organizations like Meredith Corporation exceed these returns. Workplace wellness is one of the best starting places for community sustainability. Healthier workplaces help build healthier communities.

Whole Foods shapes its wellness program with corporate values

Whole Foods is an organic food market headquartered in Austin, Texas with more than 91,000 workers. Employees can receive up to $1800 a year to cover the cost of health insurance deductions and out-of-pocket expenses (1). Whole Foods offers week-long Total Health Immersion programs that include lectures from nutritionists.

The personal wellness mission extends to customers as well. Their organic food selection is high-quality. Organics are key to avoiding hormonal imbalances associated with processed foods. The wellness program includes community outreach. Whole Foods philosophy on wellness includes the donation of personal paid vacation time to other employees who need an extra leave in times of sickness or personal hardship. Whole Foods also gives 5% of after-tax profits back to the community in which its employees live and work. Community investments such as this are exactly the type of business-community interaction that creates a healthy community.

1.   Whole Foods Market. (n.d.). About our benefits. Retrieved from http://www.wholefoodsmarket.com/careers/about-our-benefits

How churches can contribute to a wellness movement

It is advantageous for the faith community to be involved in wellness because churches are well suited for this kind of activity. Churches naturally include the community aspects of the Daniel Plan such as faith, focus, and friends that make up essential components non-physical health. The Daniel Plan is transferable to the wider national and international community as well. As more churches become involved in wellness, they can first be part of local wellness movements that help their communities become more sustainable and then join with the wider wellness movement.

The faith chapter in the Daniel Plan emphasizes (1):

- How substituting prayer for worry can be a great stress reliever

- How we can't recover our health alone. Faith connects us to a power beyond ourselves and connects us with others

- How faith helps us change the underlying beliefs that make us unwell

- How faith connects us to the healing power of unconditional love

1. The Daniel Plan. (n.d.). Success stories. Retrieved from http://www.danielplan.com/

15

ADVANTAGES OF WORKPLACE WELLNESS FOR EMPLOYERS AND EMPLOYEES

WORKPLACE WELLNESS (WW) has personal and employer benefits. Yet only 7% set up effective WW programs. When employers hear about the potential return on investment, some rush to set up a WW program. This rushing usually sets the wrong course because the wellness activities are not based on a solid baseline of personal wellness data. WELCOA has established the 7 Benchmarks of successful WW programs to ensure the development of effective, results-oriented programs instead of ineffective, activity-oriented programs (1).

What are the three essential cost areas to employers related to poor health?

- *Healthcare:* Employers pay more for insurance premiums and worker's compensation for obese employees

- *Absenteeism:* Lost wages is the cost to the employee and work not completed is a cost to the employer. Obese employees miss more days at work

- *Reduced productivity:* Obese employees work at less than full capacity

Employer Perspective

- Over 90% of employers believe that WW programs:
  - Reduce health care costs
  - Reduce absenteeism
  - Increase morale
  - Increase productivity
  - Increase retention

Financial incentives: Direct financial incentives for wellness do not occur at a significant level outside of participation in an established WW

> Healthy lifestyle cuts individual lifetime healthcare costs in half.

program. However, the healthcare savings from reversing T2D and maintaining health are very significant. As mentioned, the potential personal savings from reversing T2D is at least 50%. Healthy lifestyle cuts individual lifetime healthcare costs in half. (2) This long-term savings in health care costs is much greater than direct financial incentives provided by a large employer. Thus, employees without a workplace wellness program are not necessarily at a significant financial disadvantage overall. Becoming and staying well can save more than any workplace insurance incentive. Employees are also likely to save large medical payments on hospitalization costs associated with preventable lifestyle habits such as smoking, overeating, and physical inactivity. If a WW place wellness program is available, a participant can add to their savings through:

- Health insurance premium savings

- Health monitoring costs

- Cost of a fitness center pass
1. WELCOA. (n.d.). Capturing CEO support. Retrieved from https://www.welcoa.org/resources/capturing-ceo-support-classic-edition/

2. How healthcare impacts community sustainability [Interview by T. Schierer]. (2016, December 28). Interview with Dr. Mike Roizen at the Cleveland Clinic

Healthcare costs to employers

Cost of overweight and obese employees to employers: Healthcare costs for being overweight and obese are very similar. About 12% of total healthcare costs are obesity-related (1). Related behaviors increase the cost to about 40%. Adding smoking brings the total healthcare costs to about 70% (1,2).

> 70% of employer healthcare costs are preventable.

Employer health care cost per employee for overweight and obese employees: Per capita cost is $1429–$2741 more per year than normal-weight people. For surgeries, it costs $1,200 more to treat an obese person than a person who maintains a healthy weight who has the same condition—even though it may not be an obesity-related condition. Obese people have more complications associated with surgery, and it's more difficult to do surgery on obese patients (3).

How employers can estimate the cost of overweight and obese employees

(Total annual health care costs for the year)(0.12) = obesity cost to employer

Healthcare costs to employers (1,2)	
Overweight and obesity	12% of total health-care costs
Cost of physical inactivity	15% total healthcare costs
Overweight and obesity and inactivity	27% of total health-care costs
Obesity, poor nutrition, and inactivity employees	35–40% of total health-care costs
Obesity, poor nutrition, inactivity, and tobacco use	65–70% of total health-care costs
At least 65% of health care claim costs are attributable to lifestyle	

1. Hunnicutt, D. (2007). Collecting data to drive health efforts. Absolute Advantage, 6(4), Letter from the executive editor. Retrieved from https://www.welcoa.org/wp/wp-content/uploads/2014/06/aa_collectingdata.pdf

2. Capital Crossroads. (n.d.). Focusing on improved health for Iowans. Retrieved from http://www.capitalcrossroadsvision.com/capitals/wellness-capital/

3. Harvard T. H. Chan. (n.d.). Economic costs: Paying the price for those extra pounds. Obesity Prevention Source. Retrieved from http://www.hsph.harvard.edu/obesity-prevention-source/obesity-consequences/economic

Summary of lifestyle factors impacting employer healthcare costs
Weight
Poor nutrition
Physical inactivity
Smoking
Stress

Employer savings from reducing one lifestyle risk factor (1)

- $1,500–$3,500 savings for each person that reduces one of their risk factors.

- Employer savings from a 20% increase in physical activity is more than 20%. This is because with increased physical activity, there is a reduction in musculoskeletal issues, diabetes, and blood pressure. Additional savings would come with all of those changes.

1. Collecting Data To Drive Health Efforts. (2007). Absolute Advantage, 6(4): 1-44. Retrieved 2015, from https://www.welcoa.org/wp/wp-content/uploads/2014/06/aa_collectingdata.pdf

Large employer incentives

Because the vast majority of small companies do not have wellness programs, the clearest workplace wellness data is sourced from large companies. These employers and their incentives are an important facilitator of wellness. According to WELCOA, only recently have wellness programs at medium-sized companies been studied and there are very few studies on small companies less than 50 people.

Large employers are increasingly investing in wellness programs. As detailed in the table below, a three-fold return on investment (ROI) is possible for companies. The issue is not whether to have a wellness program, *but how to set it up*. The large return on investment for employers can be passed on to employees in the form of incentives. The incentive for employers is lower health care costs. The employer can pass the savings on to employees through a variety of incentives.

Return On Investment studies of preventative health-care at large employers (1)	
Overall WW cost to benefit ratio	1 : 3
Overall WW cost to benefit dollars for healthcare cost reduction	$1 : $3.27
Overall WW cost to benefit dollars for absentee reduction	$1 : $2.73

Large companies and organizations that have been studied for WW return on investment:

- Citibank health management program
- CalPERS: California public employees retirement system
- Bank of America
- Johnson and Johnson
- Pioneer
- Meredith
- Wellmark

1. Baicker, K., Cutler, D., & Song, Z. R. (2010). Workplace wellness programs can generate savings. Health Affairs, 29(2): 304-311. doi: 10.1377/hlthaff.2009.0626

Characteristics of Effective Wellness Programs

Successful wellness programs agree on the following:

WELCOA's benchmarks for small or large organizations

- Intensive, long-term involvement of a wellness coach and wellness community

- A program that is fine-tuned to the individual's needs and starting point

- Measurement, monitoring, and management of health risk factors

Long-term involvement of a wellness coach and wellness community provides momentum for *long-term* personal wellness.

Workplace Wellness Case Studies

Three different case studies illustrate different aspects of workplace wellness (WW). These case studies clarify that a variety of workplace wellness programs will yield results. Meredith is one

> Meredith's wellness program yielded a 4:1 return to the company in five years.

of the best examples of workplace wellness. Overall, Meredith's wellness program yielded a 4:1 return to the company in five years. The Meredith case study highlights how to increase participation rates and how to build a results-oriented program.

Meredith (1)

According to WELCOA, "Meredith is one of the nation's leading media and marketing companies with more than 3,000 employees operating in locations spread across the country. In 2011, Meredith won WELCOA's Platinum Well Workplace Award for its results-oriented wellness program."

Meredith established effective health metrics to help monitor and maintain the success of their program. The key to Meredith high participation rates is their participation-dependent reimbursement program which is summarized below. Employees are reimbursed 100% for health club memberships if they visit the health club 100 or more visits per year. In addition, employees receive lower health insurance rates for employees participating in workplace wellness.

Participation-dependent reimbursement of health club membership
100 or more visits/year=100% reimbursement
75 or more visits/year = 75% reimbursement
50 or more visits/year = 50% reimbursement
25 or more visits/year = 25% reimbursement

Savings to Meredith from workplace wellness (2006-2011): $10 million

Return on workplace wellness investment to Meredith: 4:1

Meredith participation rates	
Year	Participation rates
2007	74.8%
2009	86.5%
2011	92.9%

Participation rates are high because:

- Financial incentives are significant
- Wellness activities are fun, motivating, and inspirational
- Website automation maximizes convenience for participation

Why are participation rates important? Wellness programs such as Meredith's demonstrate the high return on investment associated with high participation. The number of employees participating in wellness and the extent of their participation both contribute to wellness savings. High participation means high savings and higher organizational wellness.

Question: What incentives would help you participate in workplace wellness?

1. A WELCOA Case Study. (2014). Wellness Council of America. Retrieved 2015, from https://www. welcoa.org/wp/wp-content/uploads/2014/06/ welcoa_case_study-meredith.pdf

Pioneer (1)

Pioneer illustrates results from a long-term, early adopter program. Pioneer is an early adopter of WW, having a program over 35-years-old. They received WELCOA's Platinum Award for WW. Pioneer identified effective risk factors and quantitated them to measure their wellness program results. The usefulness of this measurement system is Illustrated in the table below.

Costs to Pioneer	
Total Healthcare Costs	$19,136,500
Cost per risk factor	1 risk factor, Average claim, $669 6 risk factors, Average claim, $2300
Cost of wellness program	$425,000

Health parameters tracked included vitals, fitness participation, health information service participation, and telephonic lifestyle management participation. As an organization, Pioneer tracks the participation rate, demographics, health status improvement, member satisfaction, and cost/benefit threshold.

Question: What about these health metrics make them effective?

Pioneer's WW program covers all preventative exams. To assist in biometric screening, Pioneer has a self-checking station for blood pressure, pulse, and BMI. When Pioneer graphed its healthcare costs over time, they found a linear increase in health care costs in exact correlation with the timing of the type 2 diabetes epidemic. Accordingly, Pioneer has a diabetes program for at-risk employees.

Participation Rate
Screening: HealthCounts Screening program: 65–75% participation over 25 years
Exercise: Increase in exercise participation from 28% to 63% (1994–2003)

Savings to employees
$434 average savings to employee premiums per year

Another important highlight of Pioneer's program is the effectiveness of specific external programs for augmenting workplace wellness. Significant health improvements were obtained for one specific initiative promoted by Pioneer's WW program through the Iowa Heart Center. It was the Ornish program for reversing heart disease. Ornish program highlights are found in the table below.

Health improvements for the Ornish program for reversing heart disease	
Decreased LDLs	24%
Decreased depression	22%
Decreased stress	42%

1. WELCOA. (n.d.). Pioneer Hi-Bred International, Inc. Case Study. Retrieved July 15, 2017, from https://www.welcoa.org/resources/ pioneer-hi-bred-international-inc-case-study/

State of Iowa

State of Iowa wellness incentive program (1)	
# of participants	3700
Who administers the program	Wellmark in partnership with WebMD
Health insurance premium incentive	$90/month = $1080 per year
How does the State of Iowa wellness incentive program work?	
Wellness program requirements	Biometric screening for height, weight, waist size, blood pressure reading and a basic blood screening
	Online health assessment
	10 coaching calls with a WebMD health coach/ participants are selected
	Apply during the specified enrollment period
Wellness program confidentiality	Information is kept confidential
Wellness program options	Can be completed during work time

	Open to those not enrolled in health insurance
	Screening options: HyVee, worksite, doctor office, home test

Health outcomes are not a requirement. A lack of outcomes is needed for some exceptional cases in which injuries inhibit or prevent exercise and other exceptions. However, it is probably a disadvantage to those capable of full engagement in wellness. Reducing risk according to biometrics is one of the main purposes of results-oriented wellness programs (2).

1. Healthy Opportunities. (2014). Healthy opportunities: 2015 wellness program. Retrieved from https://das.iowa.gov/sites/default/files/hr/wellness/health-opp_wellness_prg/FAQ_HealthyOpp_14-0715.pdf

2. WELCOA. (n.d.). Capturing CEO support. Retrieved from https://www.welcoa.org/resources/capturing-ceo-support-classic-edition/

16

OPPORTUNITIES FOR ESTABLISHING EFFECTIVE WORKPLACE WELLNESS

WORKPLACE WELLNESS (WW) can be the most time-saving way to maintain gains in physical health. Every employee who has access to a workplace fitness facility can take full advantage of the cost savings it provides in gym fees and insurance benefits.

Workplace wellness has obvious benefits for business owners as well. The majority of large companies are aware of the financial and health benefits of WW programs. However, according to Wellness Councils of America (WELCOA), only 7% of companies have set up an effective program that includes the 7 Benchmarks necessary for significant results. Most companies have activity centered programs that do not have high-level impacts on employee and company health. Thus, there remains an overwhelming need for effective wellness programming.

You have an exciting opportunity to affect the lives of many people by creating awareness of the available resources to implement WW effectively and finding a way to become involved in helping a WW program initiate a results-oriented program. It may not occur overnight, but everyone has contact with some type of opportunity to improve workplace wellness.

> Only 7% of companies have set up an effective wellness program that includes the 7 Benchmarks necessary for success.

How many employers offer wellness programs?
51% of all companies with over 50 employees (1)
15% of all Iowa employers (2)
7% of all employers offer a results-oriented WW program (3)

1. Mattke, S., Liu, H., Caloyeras, J. P., Huang, C. Y., Van Busum, K. R., Khodyakov, D., & Shier, V. (2013). *Workplace wellness programs study: Final report*. Arlington, VA: Rand Corporation. Retrieved from http://www.dol.gov/ebsa/pdf/workplacewellnessstudyfinal.pdf

2. Capital Crossroads. (n.d.). Focusing on improved health for Iowans. Retrieved from http://www.capitalcrossroadsvision.com/capitals/wellness-capital/

3. WELCOA. (n.d.). Capturing CEO support. Retrieved from https://www.welcoa.org/resources/capturing-ceo-support-classic-edition/

How to establish an effective Workplace Wellness program

Resources for employer setup of wellness programs

WELCOA's model for successful setup of workplace wellness (WW) for large organizations (1): The WELCOA has studied and promoted the efforts of America's Healthiest Companies for over 20 years. During that period, WELCOA developed its patented Well Workplace process. WELCOA asserts that a wellness program cannot produce results in the absence of these 7 Benchmarks for Success. The 7 Benchmarks were formulated based on studies of successful WW programs. The benchmarks are designed to be implemented in order.

Benchmark #1 - Capturing CEO Support: Few WW programs have contained costs and improved employee health that don't have strong senior level support.

Benchmark #2 - Creating Cohesive Wellness Teams: "Teams are essential to building great wellness programs because they help to distribute the responsibility for wellness." A diverse team ensures that the wellness program will continue if the lead person leaves.

Benchmark #3 - Collecting Data To Drive Health Efforts: The team's first and primary responsibility is to collect baseline data upon which a measured program can be based. The data is collected using corporate culture audits, health risk appraisals, and interest surveys. This data is extremely important because it will reveal the specific areas of need and levels of interest within the organization.

Benchmark #4 - Carefully Crafting An Operating Plan: Baseline data is used to develop an operating plan for wellness within the organization. This operating plan will guide the company's efforts and investments in workplace wellness.

Benchmark #5 - Choosing Appropriate Interventions: The first four benchmarks serve as the foundation for choosing and implementing the appropriate health and productivity interventions. According to WELCOA's David Hunnicutt, the baseline data makes health intervention choices obvious. These interventions will most likely include tobacco cessation, physical activity, weight management, and stress management. They also may include fatigue management and ergonomics—depending on what the company's data reveals.

Benchmark #6 - Creating A Supportive Environment: A supportive environment is necessary to facilitate employee efforts to lead healthier lives. Physical wellness is difficult to maintain. People give up without support. Environmental interventions may take the form of policies, physical modifications, rewards, and incentives. One example is the removal of pop machines or placing them in inconvenient locations.

Benchmark #7 - Carefully Evaluating Outcomes: The final benchmark in the Well Workplace model is carefully measuring and evaluating participation, participant satisfaction, behavior modification, and cost containment. Companies such as Meredith have had outstanding success in measuring physical health risk factors and using the risk factor data to improve health through their WW program.

1. Hunnicutt, D. (2006). WELCOA's 7 benchmarks of success. *Absolute Advantage*, 6(1), Letter from the executive editor. Retrieved from https://www.welcoa.org/wp/wp-content/uploads/2014/06/aa_6.1_novdec061.pdf

Setup of WW for small organizations (1)

Small businesses make up more than 50% of the US workforce, but most small businesses do not have workplace wellness programs (1). Wellness improvements in the small business population can have a very significant impact on community and personal sustainability. Personal wellness, in turn, "is an important driver of organizational success." Small business wellness programs require more fine-tuning of the program to fit the unique characteristics of the company than for medium and large businesses.

WELCOA has initiated a study of best practices for small business workplace wellness. Small businesses operate much differently than large companies. These differences must be considered in setting up and administering a wellness program. Best practices for setting up workplace wellness for small business are as follows:

CEO Support: A letter from the CEO to the employees helps them better understand company or organizational support.

Appoint a Company Wellness Leader: A team approach does not work well with small business. A better alternative is an administrative assistant, an employee who is passionate about wellness.

Assess Employee Interest: A survey works well to determine interest level for different wellness programs options.

Conduct Health Screening: A regular screening that includes blood pressure, BMI, cholesterol, and blood glucose establishes the baseline level of health risk for each employee.

Implement an Incentive Campaign: An annual physical activity campaign works very effectively to initiate exercise habits if they are fun for participants and easy to implement.

Lunch 'n Learns: Cooking demonstrations consistently work well. Successful wellness programs use a variety of information sources to educate their employees. Implementation of the information is facilitated by making it simple and including fun when possible.

Establish A Wellness Lending Library: A good library includes medical self-care books, health magazines, instructional DVDs, audio books, and a variety of newsletters, pamphlets, and behavior change guides. Placing the lending library in a commonly traveled spot, with comfortable chairs and good lighting, increases the chances that the information is read.

Disseminate a Quarterly Newsletter: An effective newsletter will cover a variety of topics like physical activity, weight management, stress reduction, tobacco cessation, and medical self-care. In addition, full-color and ease of reading contribute to newsletter effectiveness. Health quizzes and contests help increase employee engagement.

Implement Healthy Policies into the Employee Policy Manual: Policies include mandating a tobacco-free workplace, promoting an alcohol/drug-free environment, requiring seatbelt use by all, and formulating safety/emergency procedures in the event of a disaster.

Leverage Community Resources: Establish a listing of health-promoting events each month—events such as fun-runs, health fairs, and educational seminars. These can be promoted and communicated to your employees.

1. WELCOA. (n.d.). Wellness for small business. Retrieved from https://www.welcoa.org/services/build/wellness-small-business/

Exercise: Workplace wellness (WW) outreach and transformation

If you're working for an employer with a WW program, talk to those leading the program.

- Whether you are an employee or employer, does your WW program follow WELCOA's 7 benchmarks?

If results are not tracked, or the program's participation and results are low impact, you have an opportunity to make a difference.

> There are many opportunities for you to make a difference in your employer's wellness program.

Review WELCOA's 7 benchmarks on how to gain CEO support and consider if you could become part of an initiative to improve WW for your employer.

What kind of impact could you have at your employer if you became involved in creating a results-oriented program? Prioritize two action steps and consider their potential impact. If you need extra room to describe your action steps, use the space below the table.

Existing WW program: Impact on company and employee health			
	Action 1	**Action 2**	**Specific Impact**
Physical health			
Financial health			

Vocational health			
Emotional health			
Mental health			

____

____

____

____

____

____

____

____

If your workplace doesn't have a wellness program, what kind of specific impacts could you have? Review WELCOA's 7 benchmarks (WELCOA, 2015) on how to gain CEO support and consider if you could become part of an initiating WW at your organization. What kind of impact could you have at your employer if you became involved in creating a results-oriented program? Prioritize two action steps and consider their potential impact.

Starting a WW program: Impact on company and employee health			
	Action 1	**Action 2**	**Specific Impact**
Physical health			
Financial health			
Vocational health			
Emotional health			
Mental health			

Building a workplace wellness community

The best way to begin your efforts to help your company is to help yourself become healthier. Use your company's wellness facility to begin your outreach. Positive personal stories of wellness transformation can help others become involved in wellness. Those who are not physically healthy are probably the most important members of a wellness effort. When people who need physical wellness see others like them participating in a WW program, it creates an atmosphere for broad participation. Create a welcoming environment for those who need physical wellness.

Exercise: How to utilize wellness strengths and weaknesses

1. Review each area of health and record whether it is a personal strength or a weakness.

Wellness strengths and weaknesses	
Area of health	**Weakness or Strength**
Spiritual	
Relational	
Emotional	
Mental	
Vocational	
Physical	
Financial	

2. Use the following table to identify areas where you need help and where you can help others. Type "can help others" or "need help" in the right-hand column.

Wellness outreach	
Area of health	**Can help others / need help**
Spiritual	
Relational	
Emotional	
Mental	
Vocational	
Physical	
Financial	

Small business wellness opportunities

Even though workplace wellness data has been collected almost exclusively from large employers, small employers actually present the biggest opportunities.

- Helping small business owners and employees with wellness represents the biggest need in WW

- The biggest needs can turn into the biggest opportunities

Small business makes up over 99% of the total number of businesses. Consider the following statistics from the small business administration for the U.S.:

Small businesses are (1):

- 99.7 percent of U.S. employer firms
- 64 percent of net new private-sector jobs
- 49.2 percent of private-sector employment

> Small businesses represent the biggest opportunities for workplace wellness programs.

As mentioned, very few small businesses have wellness programs, and very few small business wellness programs have been studied. Small business represents a wide open opportunity for wellness.

Helping small business owners and employees with wellness represents a bigger need than for large employers (2):

- The majority of medium to large employers have workplace wellness: 56%
- Few small companies have workplace wellness: 11%

1. SBA Office of Advocacy. (2012). Frequently asked questions: Advocacy: The voice of small business in government. Retrieved from https://www.sba.gov/sites/default/files/FAQ_Sept_2012.pdf

2. Lind, D. (2017). Iowa 2016 Employer Benefits Study. *David P. Lind Benchmark*. Retrieved from https://dplindbenchmark.com/

Is workplace wellness worth trying?

Workplace wellness is a long-term initiative. A large number of businesses have had poor experiences with workplace wellness because of high expectations and low results. Yet workplace wellness benefits are being realized by companies whose leadership and employees buy in fully to long-term participation. For example, Meredith Corporation now has a 98% participation in its wellness program (1) which has yielded a 4:1 return on their investment (2). The potential impact of workplace wellness is very high due to the high levels of chronic disease and high associated costs. This potential extends to every business that wants to lower healthcare costs and increase employee health.

Ending workplace wellness due to a bad experience damages long-term health of the company because of the long-term health insurance cost trends. Since 2001, approximately 80% of all Iowa employers offering

> 80% of all Iowa employers who offer health insurance to their employees had increases in health insurance costs every year since 2001

employees health insurance experienced annual increases in health insurance costs (3).

- Average cost increase = 11%

Consistent long-term trends won't likely change unless a consistent long-term effort is made to address cost drivers. Workplace wellness is worth trying again and investing in long-term because:

- The savings opportunity from workplace wellness will remain as long as insurance costs continue to rise.

- Because the paths to lower healthcare costs are known, no medical or technological breakthroughs are necessary.
  - Results-oriented workplace wellness programs have high success rates (welcoa.org)
  - High-level, long-term participation is possible.

1. Schierer, T. (2016) Tim O'Neil explains the keys to workplace wellness success [Video file]. Retrieved from https://vimeo.com/158077843

2. WELCOA. (n.d.). Meredith Corporation shares the secrets to its wellness program success. Retrieved from https://www.welcoa.org/resources/meredith-corporation-shares-secrets-wellness-program-success/

3. Lind, D. (2017). Iowa 2016 Employer Benefits Study. *David P. Lind Benchmark*. Retrieved from https://dplindbenchmark.com/

Exercise: Wellness for small business

1. Do you know a small business owner, or are you a small business owner? Fill in the information in the Wellness Facility Availability table.

Wellness Facility Availability		
Name	**Employer**	**Facility availability Y or N**
1.		
2.		
3.		

2. Does a wellness program exist at this business/ these businesses?

3. How can you help create wellness program awareness?

____

____

____

____

____

____

4. If you are mentoring someone who does not have a WW program, discuss wellness facility options with them and list them below. What facilities best meet their health needs? Fill in the Wellness Facility Options table.

Wellness Facility Options			
First Name	Option 1	Option 2	Option 3

17
HOW TO MAXIMIZE WORKPLACE WELLNESS

CONSIDER THE VALUE of the various investments in the exercise below:

Exercise: Wellness investment perspective

Cultural expectation on investment		
	Cultural expectation on spending (Free or paid)	Cultural perception
Food	Paid but food should be cheap	Cooking takes too much time

Car	paid	Increased status with price
House	paid	Increased status with price
Jewelry	paid	Increased status with price
Spiritual health	Free/ Reluctant investment	Status not typically associated with price
Physical health	Free wellness program expected	Status not typically associated with price
Mental health	Typically Reluctant investment	Status not typically associated with price
Emotional health	Typically Reluctant investment	Status not typically associated with price
Relational health	Typically Reluctant investment	Status not typically associated with price
Vocational health	Investment justified	Increased status with price if it pays off
Financial health	Mixed responses	Increased status with price if it pays off

Return on investment	
Food	Two-fold increase in life-time healthcare savings for healthy food
Car	Financial loss guaranteed for all but the top cars
House	Depends on the market
Jewelry	Financial loss guaranteed for all but top specimens
Spiritual health	Increased return with increased quality of investments
Physical health	Increased return with increased quality of investments
Mental health	Increased return with increased quality of investments
Emotional health	Increased return with increased quality of investments
Relational health	Increased return with increased quality of investments
Vocational health	Increased return with increased quality of investments
Financial health	Depends on the market

Buyer's remorse or Investment justified	
Car	Buyer's remorse: purchase not justified by return on investment
House	Investment justified by the market
Jewelry	Buyer's remorse: purchase not justified by return on investment
Spiritual health	Investment justified
Physical health	Investment justified
Mental health	Investment justified
Emotional health	Investment justified
Relational health	Investment justified
Vocational health	Investment justified
Financial health	Investment justified

Americans spend about half of their food budget eating out (1) and almost $3000 per year on entertainment (2). We are continually exposed to advertising that suggests that purchases of expensive cars, houses, fast food, and entertainment will make us happy.

1. Eat REAL. (n.d.). Find delicious, certified, REAL food. *United States Healthful Food Council.* Retrieved from http://ushfc.org/about/#fancy-form-delay

2. Tseng, N. (2003). Expenditures on entertainment. *Consumer Expenditure Survey Anthology,* 73-77. Retrieved from https://www.bls.gov/cex/anthology/csxanth10.pdf

Consider your current possessions. How much have you spent on material possessions compared to investing in your health?

Spending Inventory	
Spending on material items	**Spending on health**
Car	Spiritual
House	Relational
Jewelry	Emotional
Equipment	Mental
__________________	Physical
__________________	Vocational

1. What new perspectives do you have on spending?

____

____

____

____

____

____

Many people are self-employed single person business entities. In addition, most small businesses would not be financially capable of a full-service wellness program. Thus, a large portion of wellness reforms will need to come from personal wellness initiatives. People must invest personally in wellness, one health area at a time. Wellness tends to be something people expect for free. However, financial investment in wellness is part of what creates the commitment level needed to maintain wellness. Studies of vocational health demonstrate that those who consistently invest in personal growth are the most likely to achieve the highest level of success. The vast majority of the top 1% of successful business owners have made a significant investment in their own growth (1).

1. Christian Simpson. (n.d.). Leading edge success strategies for entrepreneurs & business owners. Retrieved from http://christian-simpson.com/

Sustainability perspective: According to the Centers for Medicare and Medicaid, 18% of the US GDP was spent on healthcare in 2015 (1). This is the largest healthcare expenditure by any country in history (2). Researchers who study healthcare are concerned about the future financial sustainability unless workplaces take wellness to the next level. Given the sustainability implications on a national level, the government has been active in wellness education. Results-oriented wellness is an investment that has consistently paid off for business. This track record reinforces that wellness is one of the most important investments we can make.

The U.S. has the largest healthcare expenditures by any country in history.

1. Centers for Medicare & Medicaid Services. (2016). Historical. *U.S. Centers for Medicare & Medicaid Services*. Retrieved from https://www.cms.gov/research-statistics-data-and-systems/ statistics-trends-and-reports/nationalhealthexpenddata/ nationalhealthaccountshistorical.html

2. Kane, J. (2012). Health costs: How the U.S. compares with other countries. *PBS Newshour.* http://www.pbs.org/newshour/rundown/ health-costs-how-the-us-compares-with-other-countries/

Maximizing Workplace Wellness

> Only 11% of Iowa's small employers offer some type of wellness program to their employees.

Only 11% of small Iowa employers offer some type of wellness program to their employees (1). The large employers in the Des Moines metro area such as Pioneer, Meredith, and Wellmark have excellent wellness programs. Established wellness programs can effectively facilitate the physical health and maintenance. The first order of business is to become well personally. Then, one can help spread wellness to others. Employees at firms with WW should take full advantage of their companies' wellness programs and their wellness incentives. The presence of a workplace wellness program greatly facilitates the initiation and maintenance of physical wellness.

1. Lind, D. (2016). Iowa 2016 Employer Benefits Study. Retrieved from https://dplindbenchmark.com/

Exercise: Maximizing Workplace Wellness

If you are an employee, fill out the first row. If you are an employer, fill out the second row.

1. Answer yes or no to each heading. For example, if a WW facility is available, answer "yes." Does your workplace have a wellness program? If so, is it comprehensive? Does your

employer incentivize the program? Fill in Table "Availability of Wellness Program and Incentives."

2. What type of media most helps you to learn, and what type of material do you need to learn the most? Find a learning resource that you need personally or for work and fill in the table with the names of these resources. Fill in Table "Maximizing Wellness Return on Investment (ROI)." Does the ROI bring a personal reward (indicate this with a "P") or vocational (indicate this with a "V") reward?

Availability of Wellness Program and Incentives			
	WW facility availability?	Comprehensive program?	Employer incentives?
Employee			
Employer			

Maximizing Wellness Return on Investment (ROI)		
Type of material	Specific learning resource	ROI (personally (P); vocationally (V)
Reading		
Educational video		
Vocational video		
Wellness video		

Educational maximization: There are many sources of high-quality leadership, vocational, and wellness training which can enhance workplace wellness and increase productivity. Take full advantage of these materials by reinforcing the healthy messages with a different but related program each year. This strategy reinforces existing training and expands on it by providing a new source of information or training. Both employers and employees can maximize the time and money invested in wellness. Workout facilities have TVs. Use TV as a learning resource while you workout.

3. What material is relevant to your job duties and training requirements? Make a list and prioritize it by relevance and interest. Fill in Table "Adding value to vocational wellness." For example, your top 2 reading priorities by personal interest could be "The 21 Irrefutable Laws of Leadership" and "Good to Great" for personal interest and "Biosecurity Training" and "ISO 9001" by relevance to your specific job.

4. What material could enhance your job duties and training requirements? Place your top picks in Table 1 "Adding value to vocational wellness." Include your supervisor to help you determine your selection. Record any activities selected with your supervisor in Table 2.

5. What material could enhance your personal wellness? Place your top picks in Table 3 "Adding value to personal wellness."

6. What material could enhance your organization's wellness? Place your top picks in Table 4 "Adding value to organizational wellness."

7. Fill in the tables below with specific materials and become a champion of these materials to your employer and others. Google is great for finding what you are looking for. Do a Google search on your area of interest.

Table 1: Adding value to vocational wellness		
	Direct relevance to job	**Personal interest**
Reading 1		
Reading 2		
Vocational video 1		
Vocational video 2		
Wellness video 1		
Wellness video 2		
Educational video 1		
Educational video 2		

Table 2: Adding value to vocational wellness		
	Value-added activity	**Did you inform your employer?**
Reading		
Educational video		
Vocational video		
Wellness video		

Table 3: Adding value to personal wellness		
	Value-added activity	Employer informed?
Reading		
Educational video		
Vocational video		
Wellness video		

Table 4: Adding value to organizational wellness		
	Value-added activity	Employer informed
Reading		
Educational video		
Vocational video		
Wellness video		

A high level of physical health requires at least 30' exercise per day and more is better. Once a person is in good physical condition, longer and more vigorous exercise further improves their physical and mental health. Most people are reluctant to invest large amounts of time in physical health.

Work and health do not need to compete. If we watch TV during a workout or listen to music, the content can be changed to something educational, vocational, or related to one of the other areas of health. TV or music during a workout distracts us from the physical discomfort of the workout. Educational media is just as effective at distracting from physical discomfort. For those who learn better from video than reading, workplace wellness facilities can easily be set up for educational or vocational programming.

How can this benefit both employers and employees? Office jobs tend to require significant amounts of reading and training. In many jobs, both the employer and employee need to complete a large amount of reading and training to conform to job and product/service requirements. Employees typically complain about vocational training that takes them away from their main projects. Combining workouts with educational training is a way to complete training without taking time away from existing projects. One example is the Heartcare Channel.

> Combining workouts with educational training is a way to complete training without taking time away from existing projects.

http://www.heartcarechannel.com/

HEARTCARE CHANNEL PREVIEW

- Healthy living after heart attack and/or with heart failure
- Overview of common cardiovascular conditions, procedures, and medications
- Stroke prevention, symptoms, treatment, and recovery
- Managing medications
- Reducing readmission risks

18
HOW TO BUILD BRIDGES THROUGH WELLNESS

Rationale for PHC networking

> About 70% of chronic disease is preventable.

PERSONAL SUSTAINABILITY IS the foundation for every other type of sustainability. By addressing it, the foundations for a sustainable healthcare system and sustainable workplace are laid. Movements that start at the grassroots level have the power to positively motivate personal and organizational change. Participants in a movement need to understand how to network at the grassroots level. A grassroots movement is needed to help the U.S. recover from widespread preventable illness. About 70% of chronic disease is preventable. (1) Community networks can help build the kind of momentum that helps us tackle personal wellness issues.

Network building is the practical means of building the momentum for change created by movements. In this chapter, you will learn some of the key elements in becoming part of effective networks for preventative healthcare. By engaging in these networks, you will likely provide yourself momentum for positive change.

1. WELCOA. (n.d.). Capturing CEO support. Retrieved from https://www.welcoa.org/resources/capturing-ceo-support-classic-edition/

How to identify networks that promote PHC

Effective PHC networks can and must be prioritized by sustainability needs listed in the chapter describing the 50/25 strategy. The most impactful sustainability targets are as follows:

Top 4 priority sustainability targets	
Area of need	Sustainability targets
Personal health	Preventative health-care (PHC)
Community health	Leadership-based social programs
Vocational health	Leadership culture building and workplace engagement
Environmental health	Soil and water conservation

Priority sustainability networks	
Area of need	Sustainability networks
Personal health	Preventative healthcare networks
Community health	**Community networks:** NGO, GOV, BIZ **Sector networks:** NGO, GOV, BIZ **Influence networks:** education, government, media, ministry, business, arts/entertainment, family
Vocational health	Leadership and coaching networks
Environmental health	Soil and water sustainability networks

NGO: non-governmental organization
GOV: government organization
BIZ: business sector

The top networks by sustainability priority are PHC networks, community networks (community health and vocational health), and leadership and coaching networks. All of these together determine environmental health. In terms of foundational health priorities, networks that help people with non-physical health would be the top priority. However, most people are not aware of their need for personal recovery or willing to engage in recovery. For example, people are willing to admit that they need help dealing with stress or losing weight, but most are not willing to admit that they may have an addiction.

Most people have socially accept-able addictions. The food we con-sume in the U.S. is full of addictive ingredients such as sugar, salt, and unhealthy fats. We almost all give into food addiction at some level. Addictions remain blind-spots until a person comes out of denial. Because people do not change until they are ready, there are practical barriers to placing personal recovery as a top priority. However, there are ways to build bridges to participation in recovery through more socially acceptable alternatives.

> Most people have socially acceptable addictions.

Without recovery, the root causes of unhealthy eating remain unaddressed. Problems that we are not aware of or deny cannot be improved. The problems that drive behavior come from what we believe about ourselves. To begin the process of addressing these core beliefs, some type of recovery process needs to be engaged. A recovery process is a process capable of addressing the identity issues and beliefs that drive behavior.

Bridges to Recovery	
Area of need	**Bridge to recovery**
Personal coaching	Exposure to professional coaching information
Health coaching	Exposure to nutrition information
Leadership coaching	Exposure to relationship building principles

Vocational coaching	Exposure to goal setting and self-management principles

Question: In which of the above areas do you want to learn more?

There are many possible bridges to open the door to personal recovery. The examples above are starting points. Existing health coaching, leadership coaching, and vocational development programs can be links to recovery processes. Awareness is the beginning of movement toward recovery. There are informational bridges to recovery in each area of health. Effective informational bridges provide material to people in a positive way. Bridge-building material helps people get past denial which can sometimes keep us stuck for years. Denial is arguably the most difficult stage to get through. The path out of denial for me was provided by books. Reading was a very positive and effective means of bringing me to the point of realizing my need for a recovery program. The following are good examples of programs that address identity health needs:

Area of health	Informational Bridge Resources
Spiritual	Daniel Plan
Relational	Celebrate Recovery; Divorce Care
Emotional	Emotional Intelligence
Mental	NAMI
Vocational	Kary Oberbrunner

Physical	The Blood Sugar Solution
Financial	Financial Peace University

Exercise: Building bridges to recovery

1. Who do you know who has needs in the following areas?
2. What bridge can you build with the person in need?

Bridges to Recovery	
Person in need (first name)	**Bridge to recovery**
Health coaching	
Leadership coaching	
Vocational coaching	

Each time a person engages with an informational resource that exposes them to identity health, a seed is planted. Awareness builds over time to the point where change takes place.

How to build PHC networks

Many people are becoming aware of the consequences of comfort foods on our personal and national health, and they are making changes. We are still only at the beginning of a preventative health care (PHC) movement even after decades of workplace wellness and nutrition research.

Diversity in networks increases the ability to solve problems (1). Reinforcement of compatible messages regarding health by diverse PHC networks help maintain gains in healthy living and create long-term sustainability in our communities. Thus, people who promote health through the interaction of networks in each area of health take part in building an overall PHC network.

1. Phillips, K. W. (2014). How diversity works. *Scientific American, 311*(4), 42-47. doi:10.1038/scientificamerican1014-42

Exercise: Building PHC networks

1. In each area of health, who is someone you know that is promoting health? If you do not have personal contacts in health, make a new contact through a personal contact or an informational resource.

2. Could you share an informational resource with leaders you know in each area of health?

3. Fill in the table below:

Health Contact	Informational resource
Spiritual	
Relational	
Emotional	
Mental	
Vocational	
Physical	
Financial	

4. Set up a follow-up appointment to discuss the resource you shared and related topics. Continue to build the relationship by asking questions, planting seeds, and helping them with their needs.

5. How can you work toward connecting a group of contacts involved in leading PHC in a way that reinforces healthy messages? Use your creativity. For example, if you know leaders in workplace wellness in the areas of vocational (QA trainer), physical (Wellness coach), relational (counselor), and financial health (benefits trainer), could you bring them together to form a PHC wellness committee at work? A diverse team can generate creative ways that motivate positive change in the workplace. Journal out your creative way to build a PHC network below. This is one way to be part of a workplace sustainability movement.

____

____

____

____

____

____

____

How PHC networks could interact

The degree of interaction of compatible networks of people in each area of health determines the level of reinforcement for health messages. People can start with their sphere of influence and intentionally engage in activities that promote network interaction, bridge building, and reinforcement of holistic health.

Physical health is a starting point for network building since this is already an area of widespread agreement. It is a highly useful starting point for finding common ground. It is also highly relevant to sustainability since physical wellness is one of the greatest facilitators of cost reduction, community sustainability, and national financial sustainability. Physical wellness is an inherent bridge builder. Helping someone become healthier physically is well received as an act of caring. It yields tangible results that help the person feel better and live healthier. It's a bridge that creates a path to the next level of interaction because a level of care and relationship value has been established. Physical wellness activities can simultaneously facilitate the expansion of personal networks and impact sustainability.

PHC networking progression: How do networks expand and deepen? Improvement in non-physical health is best facilitated by questions. Questions can help identify the relevant areas of foundational health to be addressed. Then the path toward foundational health can be deepened by fine-tuning the person's or group's needs, goals, and priorities.

After non-physical health, the next level of networking is vocational and financial health. People entrust their finances only to those they trust. Thus, non-physical health bridges come before significant vocational and financial partnerships can take place.

Exercise: PHC networking progression

1. Start your networking journey right where you are. Through this program, you already have a peer or family you are helping with physical health. Evaluate how the wellness journey with your mentee is impacting your relationship.

   1.1. How long have you known the mentee?

   1.2. How long have you participated in physical wellness together?

   1.3. What are the best ways you can support your mentee's physical wellness journey?

2. What additional areas of health have come up in your discussions while working on physical health?

3. Has a non-physical health need become apparent? If so, what programs and resources exist that could help address the need?

Non-physical health initiatives	
Non-physical health need	**Program or resource**
1.	
2.	
3.	

4. Journal in more detail about how these programs could help your workout partner with non-physical health.

____

____

____

____

____

____

____

Example of a progression from physical to non-physical health

- Exercise together
- Wellness discussions
- Take a class together (wellness; spiritual growth; leadership training; financial class; 7 habits) that makes a difference
- Do a community outreach activity together
- Focus on strengthening your relationship by volunteering together

The example above could work as a progression. However, starter activities depend on the mentee's priority needs. There may be one standout activity, or there may be a combination of activities that work to meet needs. More likely, a trial and error approach may be needed to discover what activities make a positive difference. Classes, workshops, and self-assessments can guide the trial and error process so that it's not too random.

Higher levels of PHC networking

Mid-level PHC networking

Networking always begins with a few significant relationships. This is a starting point to expand into a small network of people. The following exercise assumes that you have an established relationship with someone involved in workplace wellness, nutrition, healthcare, or welfare.

Exercise: Mid-level PHC networking

1. Try starting with one or two people who want to make a difference in PHC. Then find new contacts who share your mission.

____

____

____

____

Group Formation Potential		
Name	Interest level in PHC (1–10)	Shared relationships?
1.		
2.		
3.		

4.		
5.		

2. What are the group priorities? For example, do relationships need to be strengthened or is the group ready to find a common agenda?

Group Priorities		
1.		
2.		
3.		
4.		

3. What are some activities the group can try? If the group is just getting to know each other, try some relationship-building activities. If the group is at a higher level, what activities are in alignment with your common agenda?

Group Activities		
1.		
2.		
3.		

4. Do the activities reinforce the common agenda?

5. Is there regular communication among group members? What is the frequency? Fill in the table below.

<table>
<tr><td colspan="3" align="center">Group Activity Evaluation</td></tr>
<tr><td>Group Activity</td><td>Reinforcement of common agenda (Y or N)</td><td>Frequency of communication</td></tr>
<tr><td>1.</td><td></td><td></td></tr>
<tr><td>2.</td><td></td><td></td></tr>
<tr><td>3.</td><td></td><td></td></tr>
</table>

Mid-level activity examples

Relationship-building activities for a single group of friends, coworkers, or collaborators

Sports

Concert

Dinner party

Examples of new projects that can be initiated by the group at work or in the community

Formation of a workplace wellness task force

Setup of a health screening

Setup of a healthy cooking demo

Higher-level PHC networking

Higher levels of networking are built by connecting mid- or high-level groups together. Mid-level groups can join to form a higher-level network, or high-level groups can take in a mid- or high-level group. Examples of higher-level networking activities are shown below.

Collaboration between multiple groups of friends, coworkers, or activists
Leaders developing leaders
Members of the group starting new groups
Networks interacting with other networks

Collaborating groups can gain familiarity with each other relatively quickly by attending meetings or conferences sponsored by the collaborators.

Network Expansion needs

Motivation: High-impact meetings can provide motivation for a common agenda.

Awareness: New collaborators need exposure to new information to increase awareness of the organizational roles and common agenda.

Diversity: Need new and diverse contacts to stimulate our thinking. The more different someone is from us, the better we prepare for a meeting with them.

Each high-impact meeting can reinforce and add to momentum. Every urban area offers a selection of high-quality, high-impact community events. Those in rural areas are typically within a few hours' drive of access to these events. Over 80% of the U.S. population lives in urban areas and has relative ease of access. Any conference that is of sufficient quality and topically relevant to the common agenda of your PHC network provides fresh starts to build momentum. For example, the following exercise could help establish a network by inviting your contacts and continuing to interact on and expand on what is learned.

1. Do you have connections among different networks?

2. Are there meetings that can bring together collaborating groups?

Network identity	Potential meetings to facilitate collaboration
1.	
2.	

Meetings assist in bringing people together for the journey, but they are never a substitute for implementation of the PHC network agenda. Each network will have its own unique mission and process to carry out their mission. The daily work and interactions of network members are where the mission is refined and implemented. Stanford's Collective Impact model is widely used as a guide for higher level networking projects.

Collective Impact

Collective Impact is a model for organizational collaboration (1). It has been a successful model for a variety of organizations.

1. Kania, J., & Kramer, M. (2011). Collective impact: Large-scale change requires broad cross-sector coordination, yet the social sector remains focused on the isolated intervention of individual organizations. Stanford Social Innovation Review. Retrieved from http://www.ssireview. org/articles/entry/collective_impact

Components of the Collective Impact model
Common agenda
Shared measurement systems
Mutually reinforcing activities
Continuous communication
Backbone support organizations

A common agenda requires that collaborating organizations have a common understanding of the problem and a common approach to solving it. Shared measurement systems ensure that collaborative efforts remain aligned and it enables the participants to hold each other accountable and learn from each other's successes and failures. Mutually reinforcing activities divide project work in a way that allows each participant to undertake a specific set of activities at which they excel and in a way that supports and coordinates with the actions of others in the network. Continuous communication is implemented through regular meetings, creating a common vocabulary, in-person meetings with top leaders, and a structured agenda. These continuous communication activities ultimately develop trust amongst the collaborating organizations. The backbone support organization is a separate organization with a separate skill set needed to plan, manage, and support the initiative. The backbone organization capability includes technology and communications support, data collection and reporting, and various logistical and administrative details. This frees the other collaborators to concentrate on the problem-solving.

Effective decision-making

"Collective impact also requires a highly structured process that leads to effective decision making. In the case of Strive (1), staff worked with General Electric (GE) to adapt for the social sector the Six Sigma process that GE uses for its own continuous quality improvement." The Strive Six Sigma process includes training, tools, resources that define its common agenda, shared measures, and a plan of action.

1. Strive. (n.d.). Who we are. Retrieved from http://striveinternational.org/who-we-are/

Potential networks for a sustainable wellness movement

High-level networks based on sustainability priorities can eventually develop into a sustainable wellness movement.

PHC networks
Community networks
Leadership and coaching networks
Soil and water sustainability networks

Each of the above networks has a high impact on community sustainability. Therefore, sustainability is the mission that unites all of these networks and gives them direction and a common agenda. Sharing a common agenda opens the door for network collaboration as described by Stanford's model.

Sustainability networks can be united by:

> The current 69% obesity rate, and associated medical problems are estimated to overwhelm the health care system and require a doubling of the tax rate.

Healthcare tipping points: Obesity and diabesity have been epidemic since the late 1990s. A future 33% rate of type 2 diabetes, the current 69% obesity rate, and other diet-driven chronic disease are estimated to overwhelm the health care system and require a doubling of the tax rate (1,2).

Top healthcare tipping point mitigator	Preventative healthcare

1. How healthcare impacts community sustainability [Interview by T. Schierer]. (2016, December 28). Interview with Dr. Mike Roizen at the Cleveland Clinic

2. PBS. (2017). A way to save money when half of all health costs is spent on a fraction of patients [Video file]. *PBS Newshour.* Retrieved from http://www.pbs.org/newshour/bb/way-save-money-half-health-costs-spent-fraction-patients/

Welfare tipping points: Dependency-based welfare systems without sufficient spending accountability could overwhelm the social program safety net. Recipient participation and payback benefits the recipient and creates more sustainable social support support networks.

Top welfare tipping point mitigator	Leadership development
	Personal development

Financial tipping points: The vulnerability of the U.S. and global economies. Any economy attempting to service a debt larger than the economy itself has entered a danger zone.

	Preventative healthcare
Top financial tipping point mitigators	Leadership and personal development
	Community development

Environmental tipping points: Climate change is leading to extreme weather patterns globally that greatly impact soil and water resources.

	Soil conservation
Top environmental tipping point mitigators	Water conservation
	Rainforest conservation
	Climate stabilization

How a sustainability movement can mitigate tipping points: By addressing healthcare and welfare tipping points through various types of preventative healthcare, significant progress can be made toward averting tipping points.

How these networks help each other

- PHC is a demonstrated way to increase workplace engagement and productivity.

- PHC has a direct impact on welfare programs by using health programs and personal development programs to transition people from a dependency-based system to a solution-oriented system.

- PHC has a direct impact on soil and water sustainability by facilitating more sustainable networks for human food production. These networks build stronger communities and conserve soil and water resources at the same time.

The purpose of the exercise "Higher Level PHC Networking" is to identify contacts from priority sustainability networks. Identify people in these networks you already know or try to initiate with contacts found on the internet. Start by finding common ground in your interests and use that as a connection point.

Exercise: Higher-Level PHC Networking

Creating contacts among Higher Level PHC networks		
	Contact	Connection point
PHC networks		
Community networks		

Leadership and coaching networks		
Soil and water sustainability networks		

Preventative healthcare is the most practical link between different sustainability priorities because it overlaps all types of sustainability directly at some level. The networks identified in this chapter will have the biggest impact on creating a sustainable future for our communities. Community impact will define their effectiveness. The expected result of preventative healthcare networks is long-term community and environmental sustainability. Health networks can be maintained as long as a common agenda exists and a successful model is followed.

19
NEXT STEPS

WHEN YOU HAVE worked hard to achieve diabetes reversal, why negate your health gains? A caring community can keep you accountable to your goals so that the rest of life stays in the healthy range.

Review of your progress

Congratulations on your progress! Each book, podcast, workshop, or course you take helps you in your growth journey. Gains in awareness are valuable by themselves. These are seeds of awareness that can grow if nurtured by reinforcement with similar messages on healthy living, taking the next growth step, and by relationships with others on the same journey. This chapter helps you review new gains in awareness and identify the next growth step in your journey. As you apply the new awareness to your life, your capacity increases.

Implementation has much greater impact than awareness alone because it facilitates changes in non-physical health at a higher level. Our actions reveal what we really believe, and actions can help change unhealthy beliefs. We can literally act ourselves into new feelings and thoughts. For example, the 10-Day Detox is an action step that can bring cravings under control, a huge step in overcoming unhealthy beliefs. Consistent action makes us less susceptible to being manipulated by our feelings. Review your progress since the beginning of the course.

> Consistent action makes us less susceptible to being manipulated by our feelings.

Exercise: Progress review

1. What gains in awareness have occurred? First, identify the general nature of the growth that has occurred in the table below:

Area of health	Awareness Gains
Spiritual	
Relational	
Emotional	
Mental	
Physical	
Vocational	
Financial	

2. What are your top 2 areas of growth? Journal about those areas in more detail below. If you need more room, by all means, add it to your full journal. If

you felt that you grew significantly in more than 2 areas, then journal in more detail about all areas of significant growth.

____

____

____

____

____

____

____

____

3. How can you nurture your new awareness? What next steps has that awareness led to?

Awareness gain area	Next steps
Spiritual	
Relational	
Emotional	
Mental	
Physical	
Vocational	
Financial	

4. Evaluate yourself in each area of health (1–10). What areas of health need to be addressed next, and what steps can you take to nurture growth in those areas?

Awareness need areas (1–10)	Evaluation of next growth steps
Spiritual	
Relational	
Emotional	
Mental	
Physical	
Vocational	
Financial	

How to maintain your progress

There are multiple health maintenance options. Each person can take advantage of their existing resources to improve and maintain health. Participants can also substitute programs that work better than their existing programs or add programs that supplement their existing programs. An example program is provided for each area of health that can facilitate maintenance of your personal wellness. If you have an existing resource that is working for wellness maintenance, record that on line 2. If you would like to research an alternative or additional program option, record your findings on line 2.

Exercise: Identification of existing resources or new resources for growth maintenance

Area of health	Existing resources or new resources for growth maintenance
Spiritual	1. Local church/ www.saddleback.com/ www.iequip.org 2. _______________________
Relational	1. Celebrate Recovery (CR): local and national 2. _______________________
Emotional	1. CR: local and national / Talentsmart 2. _______________________
Mental	1. NAMI: local and national 2. _______________________
Physical	1. Local fitness or WW center/ The Blood Sugar Solution 2. _______________________
Vocational	1. Kary Oberbrunner 2. _______________________
Financial	1. Financial Peace University local and national 2. _______________________

Foundational health

Foundational health (non-physical health) components can be maintained by participation in an ongoing identity-based, community-based recovery program. Celebrate Recovery and participation in a healthy local church can address all typical non-physical health needs. NAMI has excellent resources for any specialized mental health issues. Finally, an ongoing personal growth plan facilitates the personal growth in any area of health (Maxwell Plan).

Non-foundational health

Physical health: As mentioned, once cravings are under control, maintenance of physical health becomes easier. The 10-Day Detox is possibly the best program for controlling cravings. Ongoing physical health maintenance needs are covered well by functional medicine doctors and health coaches.

Vocational health: Because of the wide variety of vocational resources, a maintenance program for vocational health should be designed to take advantage of the abundant selections available on the internet. Survey the available resources. Each year, select a new program to reinforce what's already working. Different programs can build upon and augment one another. Fresh resources that provide instruction in a slightly different way provide reinforcement because our beliefs grow when we observe similar messages from a variety of reliable sources. New material keeps excitement in the learning process.

Annual self-assessments useful for vocational health include the Maxwell leadership assessment (www.johnmaxwellcompany. com) and Strengths Finder.

Financial health: Financial Peace University and newsletters from daveramsey.com provide an excellent resource for financial health maintenance.

Lifelong learning

There is an abundance of excellent reading resources available for all areas of health. Reading can help create awareness in any area. In order to provide adequate coverage, a minimum of one book per month reading is recommended. A starter reading list is provided below. You may already be an experienced reader with a prioritized reading list. If so, record your top reading priorities in the table below. If your reading is consistent over time, the results compound. We can't read much in a day or week, but accumulated reading over the course of a decade or more has a significant impact on your awareness, growth, and productivity.

Exercise: Lifelong learning

Record your top reading choice in each category

Area of health	Existing resource or new resource for growth maintenance
Spiritual	1. Purpose Driven Life, Rick Warren 2. _________
Relational	1. Life's Healing Choices, John Baker 2. _________
Emotional	1. Emotional Intelligence, Dan Goleman 2. _________

Mental	1. Change Your Brain, Change Your Life, Daniel Amen 2. __________
Physical	1. Local fitness or WW center/ The Blood Sugar Solution 2. __________
Vocational	1. Day Job to Dream Job, Kary Oberbrunner 2. __________
Financial	1. Financial Peace University local and national 2. __________

Lifelong outreach

Passing along lessons we have learned is essential to the growth process. Helping others with lessons we have learned reinforces the lessons.

> Helping others with lessons we have learned reinforces the lessons.

If we don't reinforce lessons learned by passing them on, we begin to regress, and our productivity is impacted.

The purpose of the outreach component of this course was to provide an opportunity for you to enter a lifelong process of outreach. Reinforcing personal growth by helping others accumulates and compounds the longer we engage in outreach.

Exercise: Identification of outreach opportunities

- What types of volunteering have you tried?
- What types of volunteering activities connected strongly with you?
- How have you helped others in your family, at work, or in the community?
- List your top 2 outreach activities and top 2 organizations that facilitate that activity in the table below:

Top outreach activities	Organizations
1.	1. 2.
2.	1. 2.

20
FOOD ENVIRONMENT AND HEALTHY FOOD POLICIES

Blue zones helps create a healthier food environment

ORGANIZATIONS SUCH AS Blue Zones have demonstrated the importance of the food environment in the diets consumed by local residents. Blue Zones Project is a "community-wide well-being improvement initiative to help make healthy choices easier." When all parts of the community participate, including employers, schools, restaurants and grocery stores, the combined contributions add up to huge benefits for the community. This combination of organizations can lower healthcare costs, boost productivity, and improve the quality of life.

Beaver Dam Community Hospitals (BDCH) was the first to launch Blue Zones in Wisconsin. A partnership between BDCH, Healthways, and Blue Zones resulted in a community well-being improvement initiative that encourages changes to the built-environment that lead to healthier options (1).

Blue Zones began as a New York Times bestseller, *The Blue Zones: Lessons for Living Longer from the People Who've Lived the Longest* by National Geographic Fellow Dan Buettner. It has evolved into a global movement that's inspiring people to live longer, more active lives with lower rates of chronic disease. His longevity study led to the development of Blue Zones wellness programs that help people adopt the longevity practices found in Sardinia, Italy, Okinawa, Japan, and Loma Linda, California.

Some of the goals of the Wisconsin BDCH partnership include:

- Reducing obesity, smoking, and chronic disease
- Connecting neighbors
- Helping people find life purpose in our lives
- Facilitate healthy community policies such as increasing the prevalence of sidewalks, bike lanes, community gardens, mobile food markets, and farmers' markets
- Nutrition education and easier access to healthful and tasty foods
- Helping restaurants offer healthier choices and driving more traffic to the restaurants that offer delicious, healthy menu options
- Wellness best practices in schools, workplaces, and faith communities

These initiatives allow people to move naturally, connect socially, and access healthy food. When we make sustainable changes to our surroundings, we can change behaviors. The benefits of wellness are especially noticed in the workplace. Healthy employees:

- Happier
- More productive
- Take healthy habits home with them
- Have lower healthcare costs
- More connected to their colleagues
- Miss less work
- Make greater contributions

Blue Zones is helping communities implement food environmental changes around the country. However, we don't have to wait for Blue Zones to come; employers and managers can initiate the changes in the list above as they become aware. All sectors of a community have an important role in driving sustainable change. Consumers and scientists appear to be driving the changes in agriculture. In contrast, a wide variety of professional organizations appear to be driving changes in wellness behavior. Lifelong eating and activity behaviors are difficult to change without a personal network supportive of wellness goals. Behavior changes also requires a team of wellness professionals who can support the new behaviors. Consumers are responding to wellness awareness slowly partly due to a food environment where simple carbohydrates self-perpetuate through cravings. Blue Zones may help speed behavioral changes through their food environment mission.

1. Beaver Dam Community Hospitals. (2016). BDCH brings blue zones project to Dodge County. *Beaver Dam Community Hospitals, Inc.* Retrieved from https://www.bdch.com/News-Press/BDCH-Brings-Blue-Zones-Project-to-Dodge-County.aspx

Iowa aims to save billions through healthy living

Iowa is aiming to become the healthiest state. The Healthiest State Initiative is designed to help Iowa become the number one ranked state for well-being as measured by the Healthways Well-being Index (WBI). One of the major incentives is saving billions in healthcare costs through improvements in the health of the population (1). This will enable the state to redirect billions of dollars currently spent on health care to efforts that will further grow the state's economy. Iowa is making progress on its quest to become the healthiest state. It currently ranks 14th (1).

The Healthiest State Initiative utilizes Blue Zones and WBI. Both are based on long-term data from large numbers of people. To determine longevity characteristics, Blue Zones takes a systematic, environmental approach to well-being which focuses on optimizing policy, building design, social networks, and human generated entities (www.bluezones.com).

Some potentially effective ways to create an environment that makes it easier for people to make healthy choices include:

- Offering financial incentives and other types of benefits at work to reward healthy choices

- Company policies

- Restaurants policies and menu

- Government policies that incentivize health food and disincentivize unhealthy food

1. Healthiest State Initiative. (n.d.). Together, let's make Iowa the healthiest state in the nation. Retrieved from http://www.iowahealthieststate.com/

How long will the low-fat pyramid impact America?

Official diet recommendations by major organizations continue to include a high percentage of grains and carbs (ADA/ AHA).

The American Diabetes Association (ADA) diet recommendations include (1):

- vegetables
- whole grains
- fruits
- non-fat dairy products
- beans
- lean meats
- poultry
- fish

Grain recommendations include: Bulgur (cracked wheat), Whole wheat flour, Whole oats/oatmeal, Whole grain corn/corn meal, Popcorn, Brown rice, Whole rye, Whole grain barley, Whole farro, Wild rice, Buckwheat, Buckwheat flour, Triticale, Millet, Quinoa, and Sorghum.

American Heart Association (AHA) recommendations include (2):

- a variety of fruits and vegetables
- whole grains
- low-fat dairy products
- skinless poultry and fish
- nuts and legumes
- non-tropical vegetable oils

"Limit saturated fat, trans fat, sodium, red meat, sweets and sugar-sweetened beverages. If you choose to eat red meat, compare labels and select the leanest cuts available." "One of the diets that fits this pattern is the DASH (Dietary Approaches to Stop Hypertension) eating plan." The DASH diet allows high levels of grain consumption.

1. American Diabetes Association. (2014). Grains and starchy vegetables. Retrieved from http://www.diabetes.org/food-and-fitness/food/what-can-i-eat/making-healthy-food-choices/grains-and-starchy-vegetables.html#sthash.fbxTpEfD.dpuf

2. American Heart Association. (2017). The American Heart Association's diet and lifestyle recommendations. Retrieved from http://www.heart.org/HEARTORG/HealthyLiving/HealthyEating/Nutrition/The-American-Heart-Associations-Diet-and-Lifestyle-Recommendations_UCM_305855_Article.jsp#.WPwX9VPyvCQ

The ADA and AHA have high levels of influence. People trust their recommendations. A low-fat diet is still recommended by both organizations. This reinforces the belief that fat is bad and that a low-fat diet is healthy. As a result, low-fat diets will continue to have a major influence. There are several reasons that decrease the likelihood of fast change in the current food environment:

- Major organizations still recommend a low-fat diet

- Most people still crave these foods

- The food industry makes major profits from processed, carb-rich foods and high-sugar foods

- Most people will continue eating these foods even if they know that they are unhealthy. Most of those suffering a heart attack do not significantly change their eating habits (1).

For these reasons and others, organizations are working to change the food environment and cultural environment. If the food and cultural environment change towards a healthy diet, the chances of more people in the population altering their eating habits improves.

1. Davis, A. (2015). Despite having heart attack, many smoke, are obese. *Gallup*. Retrieved form http://www.gallup.com/poll/186560/heart-attack-smoke-obese.aspx

How can the American food environment change?

Food environment is one of the main determinants of the standard American diet. The typical American diet consists of about 50% carbohydrate, 15% protein, and 35% fat (1). This could be a healthy list if the quality of the calories were high. For example, 50% non-starchy vegetables, 35% olive oil, avocado, nuts, and seeds, and 15% organic poultry, fish, or vegetable protein. However, the American diet is dominated by convenience food and fast food which contain starchy carbs, unhealthy trans fats, processed fats susceptible to oxidation, and processed non-organic red meat which has been linked to cancer.

The food environment is beginning to change as healthy grocery stores, and restaurants are coming to market. Previously established grocery stores are increasing their selection of organic foods. Healthy food is delicious and satisfying. Fat and fiber help us feel full. Healthy non-deprivation diets characterized by these components can compete with existing convenience foods in taste, price, and satisfaction.

Healthy choices can compete even without a price advantage. Whole Foods is a successful, healthy grocery store chain even though it remains expensive relative to its competitors. To increase market advantage, delicious, healthy food can be combined with competitive pricing and science-based business models such as Lean Startup to facilitate market expansion (2). Recommendations for eating healthy on a budget are listed by the Environmental Working Group (3). Online grocer Thrive Market is an excellent option. Thrive provides healthy organic food at rates competitive with non-organic food.

1. Last, A. R., & Wilson, S. A. (2006). Low-carbohydrate diets. *American Family Physician*. *73*(11), 1942–1948. Retrieved from http://www.aafp.org/afp/2006/0601/p1942.html

2. Ries, E. (2011). The lean startup: How today's entrepreneurs use continuous innovation to create radically successful businesses. New York, NY: Crown Business.

3. Environmental Working Group. (n.d.). *Good food on a tight budget: A shopping guide*. Washington, DC: Environmental Working Group. Retrieved from http://static.ewg.org/reports/2012/goodfood/pdf/goodfoodonatightbudget.pdf?_ga=1.172275811.1796230987.1477933614

Science-based approach to healthy restaurants

Science-based methodologies used by research institutions around the world to develop protocols and research strategies can serve as a model for the restaurant business. Some of the most successful business models such as the Lean Startup model are based on the scientific method. The scientific method can fine-tune any process. The scientific method itself is simple. It consists of forming a hypothesis based on a review of the current literature or an experimental finding, testing the hypothesis through experimentation, and forming new hypotheses and experiments based on the results. The process is then repeated until the hypothesis is fully clarified, fully nullified, or, in the case of business, a viable product is created.

Science can form the basis for the entire set of processes needed to bring healthy restaurants to the marketplace. Contrary to popular opinion, healthy food is delicious and can contain medium to high levels (25–75%) of fat. Healthy fats such as avocado, nuts, olive oil, seeds, and coconut oil need to compose a major, not minor, part of a healthy diet. As awareness of the pitfalls of the standard American diet grows, healthy fast food will be increasingly in demand and standard fast food will decline. This is already happening with soft drinks and red meat. Menu design, nutrient content, marketing, adapting to new market drivers, supply chain issues, and any other process can be determined and fine-tuned using the scientific method.

Chick-Fil-A uses science to refine its menu

Chick-Fil-A (CFA) has a large experimental facility where they test new recipes. They have been intentional about improving the health of their menu. According to CFA, "Because food nourishes the body and soul, we're seeking ways to make fast food better" by taking "deliberate steps toward simpler ingredients, like reducing sodium and removing high fructose corn syrup and food dyes in our food."

> Chick-fil-A is working with their suppliers to completely remove all antibiotics from their chicken by 2019

Other initiatives include (1):

- 100 percent whole breast meat, with no added fillers or hormones
- Working with their suppliers to completely remove all antibiotics from their chicken by 2019
- Sustainably sourced, farmer-direct coffee from THRIVE Farmers
  - Thrive coffee provides direct revenue to THRIVE Farmers' network of family farmers in Central America. Farmers can earn up to 10 times more than they could with traditional models
- 13 menu items under 500 calories, 6 grilled items under 500 calories
- Removal of high-fructose corn syrup and artificial dyes and colors from Chick-fil-A dressings and sauces
- Reduction of sodium by 8% across 25 menu items, and up to 50% on some items
- Removal of trans fats across the menu
- Removing high-fructose corn syrup from our buns (in progress)
- Removal of TBHQ from cooking oils

1. Chick-fil-A. (n.d.). Home page. Retrieved from https://www.chick-fil-a.com/

Ethnic celebrations generate opportunity for healthy food awareness

Every community has community events. These events are opportunities for wellness. The Celebration event in Des Moines is a community event that provides an opportunity for Asian cultures to share their cultural heritage. A significant aspect of this cultural heritage is food. Asian cuisines tend to be healthier than American food, except for white rice. Ethnic community events are an excellent opportunity for Americans to be exposed to healthier food choices higher in vegetables, healthy oils, and meats. Celebrasian included a wellness tent sponsored by Wellmark. Wellness events, booths, and tents help start conversations about wellness. Those conversations, in turn, can lead to changes in health habits.

Policies that encourage health

Food funding switches can cut costs and increase federal income

Openness to directly balancing the federal budget may still be far away politically. Nonetheless, strides can be made towards balancing the budget indirectly. Whenever momentum is established at the national level, the government usually takes note and is open to enacting change. One example is the recent adjustments in the USDA dietary guidelines in response to the growing momentum in nutrition research that discredited the low-fat, high simple carb diet. The current momentum in nutrition may be sufficient for initiating further changes. Research suggests that a healthy diet would probably do more for balancing the budget and attaining national financial sustainability than direct political means. Alternatively, an effective balanced budget amendment would be based on positive cost savings not negative cuts. A very significant financial boost would also come by switching funds used for foods known to be unhealthy such as high-fructose corn syrup and highly processed foods to

> Healthy diet and lifestyle may be the most effective tool for balancing the federal budget.

fund organic vegetables or other nutrition promoting initiatives. This would reduce the healthcare cost burden associated with high-sugar diets and fund nutritious foods.

Savings in health care costs realized by a healthy populace range from a trillion dollars by 2030 (1) to $2 trillion in 10 years (2). A Healthways study of the potential impact of health risk reduction and prevention for Medicare and commercial populations estimated 10-year savings beyond $2 trillion. People with high well-being cost less. The medical costs of healthy people are 20% lower than average, while people who report low well-being cost 50% more. Low well-being also reduces work performance. One analysis found an almost $20,000 gap in productivity between surveyed employees with the lowest and highest levels of well-being.

Some of the significant programs started by Healthways include diabetes care, national standards for disease management, public health programs, and non-physical health. They use the World Health Organization's definition of health: "a state of complete physical, mental and social well-being and not merely the absence of disease or infirmity." Healthways uses the definitive well-being measurement instrument in the Gallup-Healthways Well-Being 5 to help clients understand the opportunities for improvement in their populations across the five key well-being elements: purpose, social, financial, community, and physical. Then they apply their comprehensive, highly configurable Well-Being Improvement Solution to keep healthy people healthy, mitigate lifestyle risk, and optimize care. Healthways is involved in healthcare innovation, including game theory, social network mapping, community-based health transformation, and more.

1. American Heart Association. (2013). Statistical fact sheet 2013 update. Retrieved from http://www.heart.org/idc/

groups/heart-public/@wcm/@sop/@smd/documents/
downloadable/ucm_319588.pdf

2. Healthways. (n.d.). About Healthways. Retrieved from
    http://www.healthways.com/about-us

The switch from subsidizing junk food to funding health food

Dr. David Ludwig and others have been involved in the effort to change public health policies. The wrong kinds of foods such as commodities and commodity-derived products have been subsidized at the expense of public health. For example, high-fructose corn syrup has been subsidized for the pop industry. The government is supporting a very unhealthy substance to highly profitable beverage companies. Other kinds of processed foods are also subsidized for low-income residents such as energy bars, sugar-laden cereals, and sweetened juices.

Processed food has been the major determinant of many chronic disease issues for decades. Similar to tobacco use, food that is known to lead to disease, especially diabetes, should be taxed to discourage its use, instead of subsidized. Effective subsidies support what is healthy, not what is unhealthy. The proceeds from a sugar-related taxes can be invested in the development of healthy food systems. Such an investment will likely yield a high financial return from health care cost savings. In contrast, highly processed foods yield a negative return due to health care costs from diet-driven chronic disease. Because the large numbers of people suffering from chronic illness can eventually overwhelm the healthcare system, a continuance of current policies that promote and encourage highly processed foods high in sugar can literally endanger our national finances and national security (1).

The emergence of a long-term pattern of government funding for programs that are unsustainable or unhealthy is perplexing. Modern metric analysis and lean management systems could bring about highly effective and sustainable alternatives to failed social and medical programs. Some branches of the government such as federal science programs are well run because they use best practices from the business and scientific world. The spread of best practices to more areas of the government depends on leadership. Best practices will spread as far as an effective leadership culture spreads.

1.   Ludwig, D. (2016). *Always hungry: Conquer cravings, retrain your fat cells, and lose weight permanently*. New York, NY: Grand Central Publishing.

How can nonprofits channel investment in a sustainable direction?

One of the advantages of the United States is its integrated social sectors of government, business, and NGOs. It does this better than any other nation—according to non-profit experts. These different sectors can work together to create community sustainability and financial sustainability by promoting the right kind of investment. Often momentum has to build in communities before the federal sector is ready to participate.

A combination of doctors, nutritionists, and nonprofit leaders have brought awareness of the widespread implications of the standard American diet and its role in creating the diabetes epidemic. Creating awareness at sufficient levels is leading the changes in consumption. Many people are giving up trying to lose weight with a high-carb, deprivation diet.

John Robbins is an example of the impact of the nonprofit sector on channeling resources in a sustainable direction. He founded EarthSave, an international, non-profit organization as a result of public response to his Diet for a New America. The organization promotes healthy, environmentally sound food choices, independence from the medical system, and creates awareness of "the ecological destruction and cruelty linked to the production of food animals."

His son, Ocean, cofounded the Food Revolution Network in response to the epidemics of diabetes, cancer, heart disease, chronic disease, and environmental degradation (1). The Food Revolution Network has more than 250,000 members and the collaboration of many of the top food leaders. Their influential conferences are helping create the momentum needed for sustainable change.

1. The Food Revolution Network. (n.d.). Welcome to the food revolution network. Retrieved from https://foodrevolution.org/about-us/

Citizens can safeguard the economy from the debt crisis

Entrepreneurialism often begins with volunteerism. The high level of disengagement from targeted, ongoing volunteerism has resulted in some broader trends in our society. One such trend that has been discussed for decades is the future implications of our national debt. If we ignore the debt crisis, a failure of the financial system that almost occurred in 2008 could literally impact everyone. It is a massive sustainability issue.

It is widely recognized that an economy cannot sustain a debt that has become significantly

It is widely recognized that an economy cannot sustain a debt that has become significantly larger than the economy itself.

larger than the economy itself. Since 2012, when our national debt became larger than the economy, the United States entered a level of increased economic concern. If U.S. citizens remain disengaged from the issue, a tipping point will eventually arise when our economy can no longer service the debt. Entrepreneurialism is one of the ways that our economy can be diversified and stabilized to survive such an economic crisis.

It is better to begin discussing practical means of averting such a crisis than to precipitate a crisis by reinforcing the patterns that make us vulnerable to economic collapse. Perhaps for the first time in history, ordinary citizens have the tools to make a difference in the broader economy through wellness and volunteerism. Leaders in wellness, business, banking, and finance can use their high-level skills to develop field-specific safeguards for the economy.

The practicality of problem-solving instead of politics

Who has the most political voting power? Independents who want our leaders to solve problems make up 40% of American voters whereas Democrats and Republicans have about 30% each (1). This is why election results swing so often. Sometimes, the conservative-leaning candidate wins and the next election, the liberal-leaning candidate wins. People want their leaders to solve problems, and when that doesn't happen, they vote them out. An election can be won by appealing to independents on problem-solving.

Political gridlock based on special interest issues by definition does not work. The result is that our problems keep growing. The federal budget tells us what the biggest problems are:

- healthcare and welfare
- education
- national debt
- energy

What has worked:

- Problem solving
  - Common agenda problems
  - Well defined problems

A problem-solving campaign can win an election because:

1. Numbers: If the case for problem solving is strong enough, independents can unite with moderates in either party to win an election.
2. Most voters are independents who want problems solved
3. There are common agenda problems that have clear solutions that we can work on together
   1. Chronic preventable and reversible disease
   2. Education
   3. Energy
   4. Infrastructure
   5. Soil and water conservation
   6. Workplace engagement
   7. Research and development

1. Gallup. (n.d.). Party Affiliation. Retrieved July 15, 2017, from http://www.gallup.com/poll/15370/party-affiliation.aspx

Reversal rates can guide the way

> Disease reversal rates can organize and focus future medical science.

When scientists conduct experiments, they look for physical or quantitative evidence of change. Millions of different experiments have been conducted in the history of science, but they are guided by a desire for higher-level understanding of biological function or to find solutions for problems. Disease reversal rates can organize and focus future medical science. If disease parameters are known, and the disease is reversible, then its reversal can be tracked.

Reversal rates can result in the establishment of:

- A ranked list of diseases most amenable to prevention
- A ranked list of diseases most amenable to reversal
- A list of the most effective diets for specific diseases
- Approved/recommended preventative health care (PHC) protocols for specific diseases
- A reversal timetable for specific diseases
- Healthcare cost savings estimates
- A list of comorbidities that will improve with specific PHC regimes
- A ranked list of co-reversal rates for some co-morbidities (e.g. Type 2 diabetes and heart disease co-reversal)
- A ranked list of exercise protocols or characteristics that maximize reversal for specific diseases
- Identification of transition points from treatment to PHC

Research and development (R&D) in preventative healthcare is an essential part of creating sustainable change. R&D prioritized according to sustainability priorities can increase the likelihood of successful innovation.

Midwestern soil is priceless

The natural infrastructure provides basic necessities such as clean air and water, arable soil, and fisheries. People are degrading nearly two-thirds of natural capital worldwide (1). Because our ability to produce quality food depends on a supply of quality land, there's almost no price you can put on Midwestern soil. Yet we often treat it like dirt.

According to Scientific American, "A Kushi Institute analysis of nutrient data from 1975 to 1997 found that average calcium levels in 12 fresh vegetables dropped 27 percent; iron levels 37 percent; vitamin A levels 21 percent, and vitamin C levels 30 percent. A similar study of British nutrient data from 1930 to 1980, published in the British Food Journal, found that in 20 vegetables the average calcium content had declined 19 percent; iron 22 percent; and potassium 14 percent. Yet another study concluded that one would have to eat eight oranges today to derive the same amount of Vitamin C as our grandparents would have gotten from one."

Health and wellness has implications far beyond human health. It is the most influential factor on the health of the planet. How we manage ourselves ultimately determines how well we manage our resources. Environmental carrying capacity, land management, and other environmental sustainability issues are not

> Average calcium levels in 12 fresh vegetables has dropped 27 percent

concerns for scientists alone. Everyone can make an impact on improving our environment by selecting healthy, organic food, wasting less, and volunteering in their community.

1. Tercek, M., & Adams, J. (2013). *Nature's fortune: How business and society thrive by investing in nature* [Audiobook]. New York, NY: Basic Books.

2. Scheer, R., & Moss, D. (n.d.). Dirt poor: Have fruits and vegetables become less nutritious? [Blog post]. *Scientific American*. Retrieved from http://www.scientificamerican.com/article/soil-depletion-and-nutrition-loss/